I17

CHILDHOOD DEPRESSION
School-Based Intervention

The Guilford School Practitioner Series

EDITORS

STEPHEN N. ELLIOTT, Ph.D.
University of Wisconsin – Madison

JOSEPH C. WITT, Ph.D.
Louisiana State University, Baton Rouge

.

Academic Skills Problems: Direct Assessment and Intervention
EDWARDS S. SHAPIRO

Curriculum-Based Measurement: Assessing Special Children
MARK R. SHINN (ED.)

Suicide Intervention in the Schools
SCOTT POLAND

Problems in Written Expression: Assessment and Remediation
SHARON BRADLEY-JOHNSON AND JUDI LUCAS LESIAK

Individual and Group Counseling in Schools
STEWART EHLY AND RICHARD DUSTIN

School-Home Notes: Promoting Children's
Classroom Success
MARY LOU KELLEY

Childhood Depression: School-Based Intervention
KEVIN D. STARK

CHILDHOOD DEPRESSION
School-Based Intervention

KEVIN D. STARK, Ph.D.
University of Texas at Austin

THE GUILFORD PRESS
New York   London

© 1990 The Guilford Press
A Division of Guilford Publications, Inc.
72 Spring Street, New York, NY 10012

Printed in the United States of America

This book is printed on acid-free paper.

Last digit is print number: 9   8   7   6   5   4   3   2   1

Library of Congress Cataloging-in-Publication Data

Stark, Kevin Douglas.
    Childhood depression : school-based
intervention / Kevin D. Stark.
        p.   cm.   (The Guilford school practitioner series)
    Includes bibliographical references.
    ISBN 0-89862-357-X   ISBN 0-89862-236-0 (pbk)
    1. Depression in children—Treatment.   2. Cognitive therapy, for children.   I. Title.
    [DNLM: 1. Behavior Therapy—in infancy & childhood.
2. Depression—in infancy & childhood.   WM 171 S795t]
RJ506.D4S73   1990
618.92'8527—dc20
DNLM/DLC
for Library of Congress   90-3085
                                                       CIP

Contents

1

The Nature and Diagnosis of Childhood Depressive Disorders

An English teacher stops in your office to express concern about a child whose journal entries commonly center around death and a lack of self-worth. In art class, a child sketches a picture of the sidewalk he sees below himself as he peers down between his feet from the ledge of a skyscraper. The art teacher is appropriately concerned and brings the picture to your attention. A fifth-grade girl's grades drop suddenly; she continually alienates her peers and has a history of running away from home. The third-grade teacher refers Cody to you because he has been going under his desk and crying a lot. A cute sixth-grade girl who is the star of the volleyball team, a cheerleader, and honor-roll student describes herself as fat, stupid, ugly, and undeserving of friendship. A fourth-grade boy is referred to the school nurse because he always looks tired, occasionally falls asleep in class, and is constantly complaining of aches and pains. What do these youngsters have in common? They all were experiencing an episode of a depressive disorder. Fortunately, their teachers were astute enough to alert the school psychologist to their concerns.

In this book, the expression of depression during childhood will be described along with research that has a bearing on how to help depressed youths. Screening and assessment procedures that can be used by school psychologists will be discussed. It will be argued that school psychologists need to take a proactive approach to the identification of depressed children. The last two chapters of the book describe a multicomponent treatment program for depressed children that has evolved over a number of years of treating depressed children in the schools. It is hoped that this book will alert school psychologists to the growing problem of depression during childhood and that it will serve as a catalyst for promoting greater involvement in the identification and treatment of depressed youths by psychologists in the schools. Although this book provides the reader with a description of a treatment program for depression, it serves as just one part of the training that often is necessary, and ethically mandated, for venturing into the realm of treating depressed children. Additional education and supervised practical experience are desirable.

THE NATURE OF DEPRESSION IN CHILDREN

How do children manifest depression? How does one gauge the severity of the disorder? Do depressed children qualify for special education programming? These questions and a number of other related questions will be answered in this chapter. Children manifest depression in a manner analogous to adults with some developmentally appropriate differences and age-specific associated features, according to the recently published third edition of the *Diagnostic and Statistical Manual of Mental Disorders — Revised* (DSM-III-R, APA, 1987). The existence of age-specific associated features (e.g., separation anxiety) and of developmentally appropriate manifestations of the symptoms (e.g., decreased school performance) generally is accepted. However, the nature and extent of these associated features and developmental differences are unclear, and they present a question that needs to be addressed by future research. Furthermore, it appears as though these differences may be more evident as the child being considered is younger. Most of the research completed with children, including the author's, has been with children between the ages of 9 and 13. The discussion that follows is most applicable to this age group. It is believed that the discussion will remain, for the most part, true for adolescents, but it may be less directly applicable to children under the age of 8.

Through the following discussion it will become apparent that childhood depression is more than the single *symptom* of sadness. It is a *syndrome* that is comprised of a multitude of symptoms that reliably co-occur (Carlson & Cantwell, 1980). These symptoms can be divided into the same major categories of symptoms utilized to describe depressed adults, including affective, cognitive, motivational, physical, and vegetative (Kovacs & Beck, 1977). Much of the author's exploration of the phenomenological experience of depression in children has been guided by the work of Joaquim Puig-Antich. It is through the use of the clinical interview that he developed, the Schedule for Affective Disorders and Schizophrenia for School-Aged Children, commonly referred to as the Kiddie-SADS (K-SADS; Puig-Antich & Ryan, 1986), that my colleagues and I have been able to gain an in-depth understanding of the inner and outer worlds of depressed children.

In the discussion that follows, the symptoms that comprise the syndrome of depression in children are defined and described. The descriptions are designed both to aid the school psychologist with the assessment process and to help him or her to gain an understanding of the phenomenological experience of depressed youths. Such an understanding will also aid the practitioner in his or her therapeutic endeavors, since a thorough knowledge of the experiential world of the depressed child is a prerequisite for developing effective interventions. Furthermore, this understanding of depression is necessary for the establishment of empathic understanding, which is an integral component of the therapeutic relationship. An awareness of the feelings, thoughts, and behaviors of depressed children also helps the therapist develop therapeutic strategies for dealing with some of the symptoms of depression that pose unique problems for the therapeutic process. For example, anhedonia and fatigue often coalesce to create a client who is uninvolved in treatment and who doesn't have the energy to complete therapeutic assignments. Being aware of this and other potential roadblocks to therapeutic success enables the therapist to design intervention programs that circumscribe possible impediments.

In the following discussion, each symptom will be defined, the various ways that it may be manifested will be described, and case examples will be provided. A diagnostic interview has been transcribed and can be found in Appendix A. The responses of the child during the interview are typical of those reported by depressed youngsters and provide the reader with an idea of how a depressed child describes his or her experience of some of the symptoms. Since each symptom varies along a continuum of severity, the minimum point (least severe point along the continuum of severity) where the thought, feeling, or behavior becomes symptomatic is noted. It is at this point that the behavior, thought, or feeling changes from a mild, nonclinical entity to a clinically relevant symptom. Finally, when possible, the prevalence of each symptom will be noted for a sample of depressed school children and for other populations of depressed youths. The prevalence figures of the symptoms for the general school population and for depressed youths can be found in Table 1.1. As noted above, a number of the symptoms pose special problems for the therapist. They will be identified along with remedial steps in Chapter 3.

EMOTIONAL SYMPTOMS

Dysphoric Mood

The quintessential symptom of the syndrome of depression is dysphoric (sad) mood. Prior to describing the phenomenological experience of this symptom among depressed children, a couple of caveats are necessary. First, the symptom of dysphoric mood is not specific to childhood depression. Rather, it has been referred to as a "nonspecific" symptom of childhood psychopathology because it is so commonly reported by children with all types of psychological distress (Carlson & Cantwell, 1979). What may distinguish the experience of this symptom by depressed children from the experience of children with other disorders is the severity and duration of their sadness. Secondly, not all children who are experiencing the syndrome of depression manifest the symptom of dysphoric mood. In fact, research indicates that this symptom is found in approximately 70% of depressed child psychiatric patients (Carlson & Cantwell, 1979).

The prevalence of clinical levels of dysphoric mood among depressed school children can be found in Table 1.1. Approximately 90% of children with major depression, 70% with dysthymic disorder, and 40% with depressive disorder not otherwise specified (DDNOS) reported severe levels of dysphoric mood. Some readers may be wondering how these figures could be less than 100%, since depressed children are supposed to be sad. As will become evident later in this chapter, for a diagnosis of a mood disorder, a child must either report a significant disturbance in mood or anhedonia. The disturbance in mood may take a different form than sadness. For example, some depressed children may experience anger as the primary affect of the depressive disorder. Consistent with the diagnostic criteria, some depressed youths report a clinically relevant level of anhedonia instead of, or in addition to, a serious mood disturbance. Thus, a depressed child may not report sadness but reports anhedonia or anger instead.

Children may use a variety of terms to describe their feeling of sadness, including "down," "blue," "bad," "sad," "yucky," "crumby," "depressed," and "empty." Thus, it is important to gain an under-

TABLE 1.1. Percentage of Depressed Children from Grades 4-7 Who Report Clinically Relevant Levels of Depressive Symptoms

Symptom special characteristics	Major depression (n = 11)	Dysthymic (n = 15)	Depressive disorder not otherwise specified (n = 35)	General population (n = 179)
Dysphoric Mood	91	70	40	1
Quality of mood	40	27	57	2
Association	10	0	14	1
Reactivity	50	27	100	1
Morning	10	9	0	0
Afternoon	36	18	84	0
Irritability/anger	45	30	23	2
Association	20	9	37	0
Reactivity	100	9	75	4
Morning	0	9	0	0
Afternoon	60	18	75	3
Excessive guilt	36	13	20	1
Negative self-image	91	60	37	7
Feeling unloved	54	33	20	1
Hopeless	36	33	0	1
Self-pity	18	27	9	1
Aches and pains	54	67	37	8
Hypochondriasis	9	20	7	1
Anhedonia	54	7	6	0
Fatigue	73	53	31	6
Difficulty concentrating	73	60	40	4
Psychomotor agitation	36	7	9	3
Can't sit still	100	100	66	2
Pacing	50	100	33	0
Hand wringing	50	100	33	2
Pulling/rubbing	50	100	0	1
Talking	25	0	66	1
Psychomotor retardation	18	20	3	1
Slowed speech	100	33	100	1
Increased latencies	0	33	100	1
Monotonous	100	66	100	0
Decreased speech	75	66	100	0

(continued)

TABLE 1.1. (cont.)

Symptom special characteristics	Major depression ($n = 11$)	Dysthymic ($n = 15$)	Depressive disorder not otherwise specified ($n = 35$)	General population ($n = 179$)
Slowed movements	25	33	100	0
Stupor	0	0	0	0
Social withdrawal	73	27	11	1
Social isolation	18	13	6	1
Insomnia	64	60	17	4
Initial	57	66	100	3
Middle	28	22	17	1
Terminal	14	11	34	1
Reversal	0	0	0	0
Nonrestorative	42	33	50	2
Daytime	28	44	34	3
Hypersomnia	18	13	3	1
Anorexia	27	13	6	4
Weight loss	0	0	0	1
Increased appetite	9	7	9	2
Crave sweets	27	20	9	3
Weight gain	0	0	6	0
Suicidal ideation	27	7	11	1
Acts	0	0	0	0
Seriousness	0	0	0	0
Lethality	0	0	0	0
Self-damage	0	0	3	0

standing of what the child is feeling when he or she states that he or she is feeling "crumby" or "empty." The feeling, regardless of the descriptor used, may be manifested in a variety of ways, each of which varies along a dimension of severity. Specifically, the degree of severity can be gauged by the intensity of the affective experience, duration and frequency of sadness, association with environmental events, and reactivity to the environment. A number of these manifestations as well as diurnal variation in mood are associated with endogenous (more internally, presumably biologically based) depression.

The phenomenological experience of the feeling of sadness is one of the indicators of the severity of the symptom. The mildly depressed child will experience sadness in a similar manner to when he or she has experienced a loss. Children who are experiencing a more clinically relevant level of depression, and who are more likely to be experiencing an endogenous depression, will describe the feeling of sadness as something that is unique and different from the feeling they have had in the past in response to a loss such as the death of a pet. In our sample of depressed school children (see Table 1.1), a number of the youngsters noticed a significant qualitative difference in their feeling of sadness. Somewhat surprisingly, it was especially evident among the children who received a diagnosis of DDNOS and to a lesser extent among the children who were diagnosed as experiencing major depression. This more intense experience of sadness usually first appears with the onset of the depressive episode. The sadness may, in the more severe cases, be so intense that the child reports psychic pain: "it feels so bad that it hurts." Some children report that it hurts so much that they just "can't stand it." One child described his psychic pain in the following way: "It is like being repeatedly hit in the stomach by another kid while your best friend just stands there and laughs at you."

The severity of the symptom of sadness also is a function of two time variables. The first is the amount of time each day that the child feels sad. This may vary from fleeting feelings that are less symptomatic, to sad feelings experienced for most of the child's waking day. The second time dimension refers to the duration of the episode or the amount of time in days, weeks, months, or years that the child has been feeling the sadness. Thus, when the two time dimensions are combined, it is possible that the child feels depressed for approximately 3 hours a day, 5 days per week, and this has been going on for the last 15 weeks. When gauging the severity of the symptom, the longer the duration of both time dimensions, the more severe and chronic the disorder.

The degree to which the feeling of sadness is affected by environmental events is an indicator of the severity of the symptom. Less severe experiences of sadness, and exogenously based depressions, are associated with environmental events. In other words, because of the meaning the child places on certain events he or she feels sad whenever the event occurs. The events seem to precipitate the onset of the sadness. In the extreme form of sadness, there is no association between environmental events and sadness. During the more normal, less severe experience of the feeling of sadness, the child's mood also is highly reactive to the environment. The child can be cheered up by positive experiences. Furthermore, once the child has been cheered up, the good feelings remain. In contrast, with the more seriously impaired child it may be very difficult, if not impossible, to cheer him or her up once he or she is feeling sad. In addition, if the child can be cheered up, this lift in spirits is likely to be short-lived. The child's feelings of sadness return shortly after removal of the positive event.

Another characteristic of the feeling of sadness is the daily fluctuation of mood. Some children report that their sadness comes and goes or changes in intensity during different times of the day. The child may report that he or she feels worst during the morning, afternoon, or evening. If the child reports feeling worse during specific times of the day and the mood change is evident for at least 2 hours, then this is indicative of a more severe case of dysphoria, and it is associated with endogenous depression. However, it also might be indicative of a possible stressor. The majority of the depressed youngsters who identified diurnal variation in mood reported that it was worse in the afternoon or evening after returning home. This could be caused by strained family relations as well as by some diurnal variation in biochemical balances. Likewise, it might result from the fact that the children are out of school and thus have more idle time to think and get "into" their sadness and loneliness.

When determining the severity of the symptom of dysphoric mood, it is important to consider all of the possible manifestations together. Thus, if the child is depressed for 3 hours a day, 3 days a week, and during these times of depression he or she cannot be cheered up and the feeling is so bad that it hurts, this is a more severe level of the symptom than if the child were depressed for 3 hours a day, 3 days a week, but the feeling was one of mild sadness and was highly responsive to environmental events. The minimum criterion that we use to determine whether the manifestation of dysphoric mood is symptomatic is that the child feels sad (or blue, down, etc.) for at least 3 hours a day for a minimum of 3 days a week, and that the sadness is not totally responsive to environmental events.

Angry or Irritable Mood

Anger is a very common emotion among depressed children. Brumback, Dietz-Schmidt, and Weinberg (1977) reported that 88% of their depressed sample was experiencing anger. Almost 63% of our depressed school sample reported at least moderate levels of anger, whereas 45% of the children with major depression, 30% of the dysthymic children, and 23% of the children who received diagnoses of DDNOS reported clinically relevant feelings anger. This emotion has also proven to be one of the most resistant symptoms to therapeutic change (Stark, Kaslow, Reynolds, & Kelley, 1990). Thus, the symptom of anger in depressed youths has proven to be highly problematic.

Anger, as manifested by depressed children, has many of the same descriptive characteristics as dysphoric mood. Specifically, it varies along many of the same dimensions including severity, duration, and frequency, association of mood to environmental events, reactivity to the environment, and diurnal variation. Once again, these characteristics are not orthogonal but are interrelated and are considered together when making a decision about the overall severity of the symptom. Likewise, it is important once again to compare the child's current mood characteristics to his or her premorbid (predepressive-episode) mood.

The manifestion of the severity of the feeling of anger ranges along a continuum from mild irritability or feelings of annoyance to temper outbursts, to homicidal thoughts, to feeling so angry that the child "can't stand it." Fortunately, the more severe forms appear to be fairly uncommon among children in the normal school setting. We have found, however, a few children who are so angry that they often think about hurting or even killing a family member. The more detailed and thought out the homicidal plan, the more serious it is. In such cases, it behooves the interviewer immediately to contact the child's parents and to facilitate the referral of this child to a hospital setting. One very bright, depressed seventh grader reported boobytrapping his house. He took the bolts out of the commode in his parents bathroom so that it eventually leaked after use, causing serious water damage. He also reported a desire to shoot his parents and stated that the next time they pushed him too far he was going to do it. He knew the combination to the family safe where a pistol was kept, and he knew how to use it. His parents were informed, and hospitalization was facilitated.

The duration of the symptom refers to both how long the angry feeling lasts when it occurs and also to the duration of the episode or time that the child has been experiencing the anger. The feeling of anger, however it is manifested or expressed, may be fleeting, or it may last throughout the child's waking hours for days or weeks on end. The episodic duration of the symptom may vary from a few weeks to a number of years. For example, the child may have experienced fits of anger on and off since the summer of 1986. A related characteristic is the frequency of the emotion. This refers to how often the child experiences anger. Does it occur a number of times a day, a couple of times a week, or less often? The symptom becomes clinically relevant when it lasts for at least 50% of the child's waking hours at least three times per week.

Once again, if the child feels angry for no apparent reason, or if there is no discernible pattern to the anger and thus there is no association between environmental events and mood, then the child is experiencing a more severe episode of this symptom and more likely an endogenous depression. In other words, the less connection there is between the child's anger and the environment, the more severe the symptom.

In a similar vein, the severity of the symptom can be gauged by how reactive the feeling of anger is to positive environmental events. The more the child's anger can be affected by the environment, the less severely depressed he or she is. A second factor that needs to be considered simultaneously is how long the improvement in mood lasts. If it is a short-lived improvement that is followed by a return to a state of anger, then the symptom is being manifested in a more severe way.

Finally, as with sadness, the severity of anger may vary dependent on the time of day. The child may feel worse in the morning, afternoon, or evening. In more severe cases, the child may feel angry most of the time with the feelings becoming more intense during the morning, afternoon, or evening on a regular basis. Diurnal variation is considered to be present if the child's anger becomes worse for at least 2 hours in the morning, afternoon, or evening. Similar to the feeling of sadness, more of the children who reported diurnal variation reported that their feelings of anger were more intense during the afternoon or evening. In fact, very few of the depressed children reported that the feeling of anger was worse in the morning, whereas 60% with major depression, 18% with dysthymia, and 75% with DDNOS reported that their anger was worse in the afternoon or evening.

Anhedonia

Anhedonia is the loss of the pleasure response. The child no longer derives pleasure from activities or events that he or she enjoyed prior to the onset of the depressive episode. A reduction in both the number of activities that the child finds pleasurable and the amount of pleasure that the child derives from them is observed. The child now feels bored, uninterested, or as if he or she is just going through the motions. The child does not have as much fun in previously enjoyed activities. For example, a 14-year-old girl described her loss of pleasure in the following way. On being voted by her peers to be one of the school cheerleaders (an achievement she had placed a great deal of importance in prior to the depressive episode), she stated that it didn't mean anything to her. She just stood on stage and watched the other girls get excited, but she didn't feel anything. She didn't feel excited or even happy. She simply was there and did what she thought she was supposed to do.

The symptom of anhedonia becomes clinically relevant when the child is bored over half of his or her waking hours or when the child no longer derives as much pleasure from over half of the activities that he or she enjoyed prior to the depressive episode. The most severe expression of the symptom is the complete inability to derive pleasure from anything. As will become evident later, anhedonia is one of the primary diagnostic symptoms of depressive disorders. Carlson and Cantwell (1979) reported that 67% of their depressed sample reported anhedonia, whereas it was much less common (23%) among a psychiatric control group. In our school sample, 54% of the children with major depression reported clinically relevant levels of anhedonia, whereas anhedonia was relatively uncommon among the dysthymic youngsters and children who reported DDNOS.

Weepiness

Depressed children tend to cry more, and their crying commonly is unrelated to environmental events. They also tend to exhibit a lowered threshold for negative environmental events. A broader range of lower-level events trigger tears. It is not uncommon for a depressed youngster to cry through the diagnostic interview. In general, the severity of the symptom parallels the amount of crying that the child does. However, the extreme of this symptom is a paradox; the child feels like crying a lot of the time but cannot do it. Crying is considered to be symptomatic when the available information indicates that the child has been crying at least two times a day for a minimum of 4 days of the week.

Loss of Mirth Response

The depressed child is less capable of responding to humor. The child does not find many things to be funny. He or she rarely laughs or even smiles in response to a joke or humorous situation. These children respond with a deadpan look to things that other children would at least smile about. This behavior is considered to be symptomatic when the child reports a noticeable change in his or her sense of humor and when the child's behavior during the interview indicates that the child exhibits a greatly restricted sense of humor.

Feeling Unloved

This symptom refers to the child's perception that no one loves or cares for him or her. It is important to differentiate this symptom from the normal reaction of a child to punishment. Children commonly respond to parental discipline with the feeling that their parents do not love or care about them. The depressed child feels this way at other times as well. Furthermore, when the child has such feelings, it may be difficult or impossible to reassure the child that someone loves him or her. In the face of conflicting evidence such as a parent directly stating that she loves the child, the child still dismisses the statement as untrue. Some depressed children become preoccupied with the feeling and belief that no one loves them. Feeling unloved becomes symptomatic when the child experiences the emotion a number of times per day and for at least 4 days per week. As is evident in Table 1.1, about half of the children with major depression, one-third of the dysthymic children, and one-fifth of the children who reported DDNOS reported feeling unloved.

Self-Pity

Self-pity refers to feeling sorry for oneself as a result of the belief that life has been unfair or more difficult or less fulfilling than that of the child's peers. The severity of this symptom is gauged by the amount of time the child spends feeling sorry for himself or herself. It is important to differentiate these unrealistic feelings of self-pity from feelings that may be based in reality. The child may in fact have led a very difficult life filled with hardships. In such cases, the self-pity only becomes symptomatic when the child spends an inordinate amount of time dwelling on his or her unfortunate situation. Self-pity was reported by less than 25% of the depressed school population.

COGNITIVE SYMPTOMS

Negative Self-Evaluations

Researchers (see Kendall, Stark, & Adam, 1990) indicate that depressed children negatively evaluate their performances, abilities, and other meaningful personal qualities. It appears as though negative self-evaluations are one of the most common symptoms of depression. Brumback et al. (1977) reported that the symptom was present in over 97% of their depressed sample of chi'dren. It was nearly as common (91%) among the author's sample of depressed school children with major depression. Depressed children tend to perceive themselves as inadequate and their performance as unacceptable, and these perceptions often persist in the face of contradictory information. Such negative self-evaluations contribute to a low level of self-esteem. Low levels of self-esteem have been reported for depressed children (Kazdin, Colbus, & Rodgers, 1986; Stark, Kaslow, Hill, & Lux, 1990). However, it is important to note that negative self-evaluations and low self-esteem are not specific to depression. Rather, they appear to be associated with many psychological disorders.

The severity of the symptom of negative self-evaluations can be gauged by the number of personal qualities, and so forth, that the child views negatively as well as the depth of the negative evaluations. The child may negatively evaluate him or herself in just one area such as performance in school, or the child may negatively evaluate him or herself in all areas of life. In addition, the child's negative self-evaluations fall along a continuum of severity. For example, a child might consider his or her athletic performance as just slightly unacceptable to totally unacceptable — which may include hatred of that characteristic. The extreme example of this symptom is self-hatred. Although this extreme is dramatic and obviously symptomatic, we generally consider a report of negative evaluations in at least three primary domains of self-description to be indicative of a significant symptom. The domains may be such things as intelligence, physical appearance, personality, personal possessions, scholastic achievement, or athletic ability.

The debilitating nature of negative self-evaluations should not be underestimated. Robbins and Alessi (1985) reported that negative self-evaluations were significantly associated with suicidal behavior. Specifically, negative self-evaluations were associated with suicidal gestures, attempts, and the medical lethality of the attempts.

Guilt

Guilt is the descriptor for the remorseful feeling that people have following misbehaving or hurting another individual. It is classified as one of the cognitive symptoms because it is assumed to reflect the child's attributional style. The feeling only follows an internal attribution for a negative outcome. In other words, people only feel guilty when they believe they caused the unfortunate outcome. Typically, a person does not feel guilty if he or she believes that someone else caused the negative event to occur. Research indicates that children who endorse moderate levels of depressive symptomatology make internal (to the self), stable (long-lasting), and global (across situations) attributions for negative outcomes (Seligman et al., 1984), and hence their feelings of guilt.

Most children experience normal feelings of guilt on occasion. The feeling becomes symptomatic when it occurs for unusually long periods of time (in excess of 2 hours per day, 3 days per week), when it occurs after events that the child objectively could not have caused, and/or when the child believes that he or she should be excessively punished for his or her misbehavior. Research (Kashani, Barbero, & Bolander, 1981) indicates that approximately 62% of depressed children report excessive or inappropriate guilt. Excessive guilt was much less common among our sample of depressed school children (see Table 1.1). An example of a severe level of this symptom is a girl who felt guilty about her best friend's death in a car accident. In fact, she didn't play any objective role in the accident. Additionally, she was still experiencing the guilty feeling 2 years after it happened. Finally, she believed that she should be punished in the form of never being able to have any friends again.

Hopelessness

Hopelessness is the expectation that the future either will not improve or will be worse than the child's current situation. Carlson and Cantwell (1979) found that approximately 70% of their depressed sample of children were experiencing hopelessness. Hopelessness was reported by approximately one third of the school children with major depression and dysthymic disorder. None of the youngsters with DDNOS reported a significant level of hopelessness. The hopeless youngster feels discouraged because he or she does not see any possibility for a solution to his or her problems. Children who are depressed and hopeless believe that their current situation is unpleasant, and they have no hope for things getting better in the future. Since the child thinks that his or her problems will continue to mount, and since he or she does not see any hope for solving them, the child may believe that the only escape is through suicide. Suicidal ideation and behavior have been found to be more highly associated with hopelessness than with depression (Kazdin, French Unis, Esveldt-Dawson, & Sherick, 1983). Thus, if the child expresses hopelessness and a fair amount of additional symptomatology as well as suicidal ideation, the youngster is at a high risk for attempting suicide. A particular problem that this symptom often poses for the therapist is that the hopeless child also does not see any chance for therapy to produce improvements in his or her depressive symptomatology. Thus, such a child may not be motivated to invest any energy into therapy.

Difficulty Concentrating

As the previous discussion may have implied, depressed children spend a good deal of time thinking about their "sorry" plight. They become lost in the negative world of thoughts they have created inside their heads. Because of this preoccupation, they have a difficult time concentrating on what is happening in their outside world. Their depressogenic cognitions interrupt their train of thought. This disruption may be minimal, such as fleeting breaks in concentration, or it may be more extreme, such as when there is a complete inability to concentrate on things even when the child is putting forth effort and the material is of interest. This problem becomes symptomatic when the child's lack of concentration affects his or her performance in school. It appears as though this symptom is fairly common among depressed youth. Kashani, Barbero, and colleagues (1981) reported that 77% of their sample of depressed children exhibited difficulty concentrating and indecision. Difficulty concentrating was very common among our depressed school children. Over half of the children with major depression reported difficulty concentrating.

Indecisiveness

Perhaps as a result of their low self-esteem, negative expectations for the future, and difficulty concentrating on one topic, some depressed children also have difficulty making or sticking with decisions. They do not see a high probability of success in any outcome, so it becomes difficult to choose one. This inability to make decisions leads to impaired school performance and greater dependency on adults for decision making.

Morbid Ideation

A depressed child may become preoccupied with death. The child may obsess about an actual death or be overly concerned about someone dying. It is natural to mourn and think about the death of a significant other or a pet. This ideation becomes symptomatic when it goes on for an extended period of time after the death or when it is not objectively probable that the individual or other living thing is going to die. Additionally, if the child becomes preoccupied with death itself, unrelated to a personal loss, such as through reading books or newspaper articles about it or by showing an unusual fascination with death as it is portrayed through other forms of communication, this also is symptomatic. If the child appears to be preoccupied with his or her own death, this may be an indication of suicidal intent. It is imperative in such situations to pursue an assessment of suicidal ideation and behavior.

MOTIVATIONAL SYMPTOMS

Social Withdrawal

Social withdrawal refers to a decline in the frequency of contact and depth of involvement with other children and adults. The withdrawn child will evidence a decrease, relative to pre-episode behavior, in social contacts and involvements with family, friends, and other social acquaintances. This symptom has been reported to occur among 67% of a depressed sample of children (Brumback et al., 1977). Social withdrawal was reported by nearly 75% of school children with major depression. It was much less common among the other two depressed groups. The socially withdrawn child, unlike the social isolate, was socially active prior to the onset of the depressive episode. In fact, the child may not like to be withdrawn; however, he or she can't help him or herself. The withdrawal may range in severity from a moderate reduction in time talking and playing with others to an active avoidance of social contact with no recognition that the other person exists. In fact, the child may play an unwitting role in his or her withdrawal. Friends may come over and ask the child to come out and play, but the child declines the invitation. The youngster also may initiate oppressive behaviors that result in other children rejecting or avoiding the child. The withdrawal becomes symptomatic when the child finds that he or she is turning away friends and avoiding contacts with children at school as well as his or her parents or other adults.

A sixth-grade boy manifested his social withdrawal in the following way. He did not initiate any social behavior at school and only spoke minimally in those situations where he had to. When he came home from school, he went straight to his room without greeting his family. Once in his room, he pulled the shades, closed the door, and then, just to be sure he was "sealed in," he took the rug and stuffed it in the crack under the door, thus ensuring that he did not have any contact with the outside world.

Suicidal Ideation and Behavior

Although suicide is rare before the age of 10, older children do think about and commit suicide. In fact, Carlson and Cantwell (1982) found that approximately 89% of their depressed sample of children reported suicidal ideation. In another study, Pfeffer, Zuckerman, Plutchik, and Mizruchi (1984) reported that 13.9% of a sample of school children reported significant suicidal behavior. In our sample of school children, suicidal ideation was reported by 25% of the children with major depression and 10% of the children from the other two diagnostic groups. None of the children engaged in clinically relevant suicidal behavior. When such a child takes his or her life, it is one of the greatest tragedies. Such an event affects more than the child and his or her family; it also impacts the child's school and many times the entire community.

One of the best predictors of suicidal behavior is suicidal ideation. Suicidal ideation is thinking about killing oneself. It includes thoughts about death such as "I would be better off dead," "My parents would be happier if I were dead," "No one cares about me, I might as well be dead," "I could end all of the suffering by killing myself," and "The only way to end it all is to kill myself." It also includes thoughts about how the child would go about completing the self-destructive act. This includes the child's plan. The critical point is that the child clearly expresses an interest or desire to kill him or herself within these thoughts.

The severity of the suicidal ideation can be gauged by the content of the thoughts. More specifically, it can be measured by the intensity of the desire to kill oneself and the specificity of the plan. The more specific, detailed, and well thought out the plan, the more severe the suicidal ideation, and the more likely the child will make an attempt. Another measure of the severity of the suicidal ideation is the degree of hopelessness in the child's thoughts. If the child does not express any hope for improvement in the future, or if it becomes apparent through questioning that the child holds little hope for the future, then this is a very severe and serious expression of suicidal ideation. The severity of the suicidal intent and plan can be gauged by another bit of information that may be evident from listening to the child's fantasies (thoughts and images) about the suicidal plan. If the act is to be carried out in the presence of others, then the intent is less severe than if the plan is to be carried out when no one else is around. If the other people (e.g., parents) are present or close by, then it is possible that the child is building in a safety net in the hope that someone will stop him or her, and the failed attempt will serve as a strong message that there is a need for help and change.

Suicidal behavior is any action taken by the child that is instrumental in causing self-harm that could lead to death or is intended to cause the child's death even if it couldn't objectively do so. This not only includes behavior that directly inflicts harm (e.g., swallowing pills) but also includes other behavior that is part of the plan and is necessary for actually harming oneself, such as acquiring a gun, hunting knife, razor, pills, and so forth. The definitive factor is that it is purposive behavior that is instrumental in carrying out the child's desire to kill him or herself. All of this behavior is very severe. However, it may vary along a dimension of severity commonly referred to as medical lethality. The more lethal the behavior (the greater the likelihood that the behavior would produce death), the more severe it is. Thus, shooting oneself in the head is more severe (lethal) than swallowing a dozen aspirin. The latter is likely to induce vomiting and not death, whereas the former has a high probability of causing death.

Previous attempts to commit suicide are another very relevant suicidal behavior and an indicator of a severe problem. Children who have attempted suicide are more likely than other children to make another attempt. The more lethal the attempt, the more serious it was and the greater the likelihood that the youngster will once again make a serious and highly lethal attempt.

Decreased Academic Performance

Relative to their premorbid behavior, some depressed children evidence decreased school performance. In fact, a number of investigators have found this symptom to be fairly common among depressed youths. Carlson and Cantwell (1979) reported that 48% of their depressed sample of children were experiencing academic difficulties. Brumback et al. (1977) found academic difficulties among 71% of their depressed sample, whereas 62% of Kaslow, Tannenbaum, Abramson, Peterson, and Seligman's (1983) sample were experiencing a decrease in academic performance. These children often appear to be unmotivated to learn. This is not surprising given the cognitive set that includes such ideas as "I'll never be able to do that," "I'm not as smart as the other kids," "I can't do that," "I'll just get it wrong anyway," "It's too hard," "Nobody cares," "It just doesn't matter," "I don't feel up to it," or "They'll just find something else to complain about." In addition, the child may not have the psychic energy to work hard. The symptom of fatigue may leave the child feeling tired, apathetic, and as if he or she just can't muster enough energy to do the required academic tasks such as completing homework assignments or studying for exams. As a result, the child's grades suffer. Decreased academic performance becomes symptomatic when any of the child's grades begin to decline by a measurable amount.

A number of other previously mentioned symptoms also compound the problem and lead to a decline in school performance. Difficulties concentrating make it hard for the child to acquire knowledge in class or through out-of-class assignments. The child may become frustrated more easily and thus prematurely give up on more difficult learning tasks. The child may be more irritable and as a result lash out at those people trying to help him or her. For example, a youngster may be having difficulty completing a math assignment. When the teacher or a peer tries to help by pointing out mistakes, the child personalizes this and becomes angry and verbally lashes out at the individual. As a result, the teacher or peer is less likely to try to give the child individual help in the future. A more thorough discussion of the impact of depression on academic performance and intellectual functioning can be found in Chapter 2.

PHYSICAL AND VEGETATIVE SYMPTOMS

Fatigue

The symptom of fatigue refers to the subjective feeling of being tired or lacking the necessary energy to pursue action. It is important to differentiate this symptom from fatigue that is objectively based on a lack of sleep or that results from prolonged hard physical or mental work. It also is differentiated from sleepiness. Fatigue refers more to a feeling of not having any energy and thus needing to rest or conserve resources, whereas sleepiness refers more to feeling as though one needs more sleep. In this latter case, the individual will take naps, whereas in the former case the individual will just sit or lie motionless. Fatigue was reported by 52% of Brumback et al.'s (1977) sample of depressed children, 73% of our sample of children with major depression, and it was reported by 53% of the dysthymic children and 31% of the children with DDNOS.

This sensation of being tired varies along a continuum of severity.

In its more mild form, the child may notice a slight decline in energy that is annoying but doesn't really result in any changes in school performance or recreational activities. As the symptom becomes more severe, it begins to impact the child's daily activities. Completing usual tasks takes longer or becomes untenable. The child may begin taking short rests during the day, sometimes even interrupting or delaying play to rest. As it becomes more extreme, the child feels tired or lethargic most of the day. His or her arms and legs may even feel heavy, as though it takes a great deal of energy to move them. The amount of time the child spends resting also increases. In its most extreme form, the child feels completely listless all day long and spends most of his or her time resting. Feeling fatigued becomes symptomatic when it starts to interfere with the child's daily activities.

Change in Appetite and/or Weight

A change in appetite may be associated with the depressive episode. Kashani, Barbero, et al. (1981) reported a disturbance in eating among 58% of their sample of depressed children. This symptom was much less common among our sample of depressed school children. The child experiencing this symptom may lose his or her appetite, or the child's appetite might increase relative to preepisodic level and relative to the child's peers. In the case of a decline in appetite, the child does not feel as hungry before and during meals, or the child may not eat as much. Once again the symptom varies along a continuum of severity from a slight decrease to never feeling hungry. Concurrently, the amount of food consumed may decline slightly to a complete elimination of any eating. This decline in appetite and actual consumption may produce a weight loss. It also may result in the child just failing to gain any weight, which also is symptomatic for a growing youngster. The child may stay the same weight for an extended period of time while he or she is getting taller and should have been gaining weight.

When assessing the presence of this symptom, it is important to determine whether the child is on a diet or taking appetite suppressants. Another confounding factor is that children will report not feeling hungry for some meals. Additional probing reveals that the child is only hungry when the meal is comprised of a food that he or she likes. Obviously this is not symptomatic. Dieting is extremely common among girls in grades 6 and up. We generally consider the child's eating to be symptomatic when there is a noticeable decline in appetite such as not feeling hungry for half of the child's meals and/or if the child reports a nondietary weight loss of at least 6 pounds or a failure to gain at least 6 pounds over a period of time in which such weight gain would have been expected.

Increased appetite and unusual weight gain appear to be less common than decreased appetite among depressed children. Some children report an increase in the amount of time they are hungry as well as in how hungry they are. They may feel so hungry that they just cannot stop eating. Concurrent with the increased feelings of hunger, the child may consume more food. The amount may be slight to unrestrained gorging. Once again, it is important to differentiate between the symptom of excessive appetite and weight gain and the normal increase that may be associated with the natural growth process. We consider increased appetite to be symptomatic whenever it is causing the child to become overweight for his or her height, whenever the ruminating about food interferes with other activities such as schoolwork or recreational activities, or when the child loses control of his or her food consumption. Parallel to decreased appetite and weight loss, we consider increased appetite to be symptomatic whenever the child notices that he or she is hungry over 50% of the time between meals, cannot restrain from eating, or has gained in excess of 6 pounds above his or her ideal or pre-episodic weight.

Aches and Pains

Somatic complaints are relatively common among depressed children. These complaints are considered to be symptomatic whenever there is no objective, medical reason for the pain. The most common complaints are headaches, stomachaches, backaches, leg pains, and general discomfort. Somatic complaints were found among approximately 50% of the depressed youths in the Brumback et al. (1977) sample. It also was quite common in our sample (see Table 1.1). The severity of the symptom is gauged by (1) the intensity of the pain, (2) the frequency of occurrence, (3) the responsiveness of the pain to treatment efforts, and (4) the degree of disruption in the child's daily activities caused by the aches or pain. The aches or pains are severe enough to be considered symptomatic when they interfere with the child's school performance or recreational activities or when the child experiences a moderate level of discomfort that is nonresponsive to self-medication and occurs at least several times a week. For example, an 11-year-old boy reported having throbbing headaches three times a week that produced enough discomfort to interrupt his ability to concentrate in school and to play.

Sleep Disturbance

Sleep disturbance is one of the most common symptoms of depression. Kashani, Barbero, et al. (1981) reported that 92% of their depressed youngsters reported some form of sleep disturbance. Although sleep disorders were less common among the depressed school sample, they were reported by a majority of the children. Problems with sleeping can be manifested in a variety of different ways. Perhaps the most basic distinction between the various manifestations is in terms of whether they produce a change in total amount of sleep. The manifestations that are characterized by a reduction in sleep are referred to as insomnia, whereas those characterized by an increase in sleep are referred to as hypersomnia. There also are a number of manifestations that are characterized by a disturbance in sleep behavior but not in total duration of sleep.

Insomnia

There are three types of insomnia that are distinguished by the point in the sleep cycle in which the disturbance occurs. It is normal for children to lie awake for a short period of time before falling asleep. Initial insomnia is characterized by an extended period of awake time before falling asleep. The severity of the symptom is dependent on the length of time it takes to fall asleep and the frequency of the difficulty. We consider the problem to be symptomatic whenever it takes the child at least 1 hour to fall asleep, and this occurs a minimum of three times a week. The longer the child remains awake and the more frequently initial insomnia occurs, the more severe the symptom is.

Children who suffer from middle insomnia have difficulty staying asleep. They wake up during the night and remain awake for some time. It is normal for children to wake up because of a bad dream or to urinate. However, children usually fall back to sleep right away. Children who are suffering from middle insomnia awaken for no apparent reason or because they are awakened by thoughts that they can't stop. Once awakened, the children lie awake and think about their sorry plight. The severity of the symptom is gauged by how many times the child wakes up each night, by how long it takes the child to fall back to sleep, and the number of days a week that the child experiences the sleep disturbance. The problem becomes symptomatic when the child is awake for at least 1 hour, 3 nights a week.

Terminal insomnia is early morning awakening that is accompanied by an inability to fall back to sleep. The child awakens unusually early, before he or she needs to, and cannot go back to sleep. The severity of this symptom is determined by the number of hours the child wakes up before he or she needs to and by the frequency of its occurrence. This disturbance is considered to be symptomatic when the child wakes up at least 1 hour early, 3 days out of the week. Of the three types of insomnia, initial insomnia was most common among our depressed school sample.

Hypersomnia

Hypersomnia is sleeping more in a 24-hour period than is normal for the child's age. This may include sleeping much later into the morning, going back to sleep after waking in the morning, and getting extra sleep by taking naps. The severity of the symptom is determined by how much longer the child sleeps than usual and the frequency of this disturbance. This form of sleep disturbance is considered to be symptomatic when the child sleeps for a total of at least 1 extra hour per day for 3 days a week.

Other Sleep Disorders

As noted above, there are other manifestations of sleep disturbance that are not characterized by a change in total sleep. Rather, these disorders are characterized by a disturbance in sleep behavior or the subjective feeling of sleepiness. A very severe and unusual sleep disturbance is circadian reversal. The child's sleep cycle is reversed. He or she sleeps during the day and stays awake at night. This reversal becomes the child's daily sleep pattern.

Another fairly common sleep disturbance is nonrestorative sleep. Even though the child gets enough sleep, or perhaps even gets more sleep than he or she used to, the child still feels tired. The severity of this symptom is a function of the intensity of the feeling of being tired, the duration of time per day that the child feels tired, and the frequency that it occurs. In its most extreme form, the child feels completely exhausted during all of his or her waking hours. We consider this manifestation to be symptomatic if the child does not feel rested on waking and feels sleepy for at least 1 hour 3 days a week. Of course, this does not include normal feelings of sleepiness that occur prior to bedtime.

Psychomotor Retardation

Psychomotor retardation is the slowing down of the child's bodily movements, speech, and reaction times. It refers to an objective, visible slowing down. The affected child may walk more slowly and appear to be slumped over. His or her arm movements to retrieve an object may be slower. In general, the child will look as though he or she is being viewed in a slow motion replay. The child may even report that she feels as though she is moving in slow motion or as if there are "weights strapped to my hands and feet that I'm dragging along behind me." The extreme form of this symptom is a depressive stupor in which the child becomes immobile. Psychomotor retardation was reported by approximately 20% of our depressed sample that were diagnosed with either major depression or dysthymic disorder. Most of these children reported that the disturbance was evident in their speech.

The child's speech may be affected in a number of different ways. First, the child may speak more slowly. At times, such children speak so slowly that it is difficult to refrain from filling in the words for them. Secondly, the child may speak in a monotone and in a low, almost inaudible voice. The amount of speech also may decrease as the child responds with minimal answers. The extreme manifestation is elective mutism. Finally, there may be extended latencies between replies to questions or even between the end of one sentence and the beginning of another.

Increased latencies to respond are not unique to communicative behavior; rather, it is a generalized manifestation that is apparent in other reactions as well. The child's reaction time in general is slowed down. This may be evident in such activities as athletic endeavors, catching a falling object, or responding to others' movements.

All of the possible manifestations of psychomotor retardation are considered simultaneously when determining whether the behavior is symptomatic. If the child's speech and body movements are noticeably retarded with marked latencies to respond, and the child does not initiate any behavior to keep the conversation going, then the symptom is scored positively.

Psychomotor Agitation

Psychomotor agitation is the opposite end of the behavioral spectrum from psychomotor retardation. In this case, the manifestations are characterized by behavioral excesses that frequently are accompanied by angry acting out. The agitated child appears to be unable to sit still. He or she is in a constant state of movement. The child may fidget, pace, rub, or pull on himself or herself or clothing, and/or the child might wring his or her hands or twiddle his or her fingers. Psychomotor agitation was reported by 36% of our sample with major depression, but it was only reported by a few children from the other depressed groups. All of the children who reported the disturbance had difficulty sitting still.

The child's speech also may be affected. It has a definite pressed quality to it as it seems to just burst forth as if the words are being involuntarily pressed out of the child. There are short latencies between sentences that may make them sound as though they are running together. In addition, the child's speech may run over that of another speaker, creating a very one-sided conversation. In its most extreme form, the child may talk endlessly with little apparent control.

Like the agitated adult, the agitated child also may be angry or irritable, occasionally lashing out at others. The child may throw temper tantrums that include shouting, using profane language, throwing objects, breaking things, and hitting either himself or herself or other people. For example, an 11-year-old girl would become angry with the slightest implication of provocation. After seeing her boyfriend talking to another girl, she proceeded to shout profanities at both of them; she kicked lockers, threw books, and banged her fists and head against the wall before school personnel interceded. She was reluctantly escorted to the counselor's office, where she yelled at the counselor and consulting psychologist. Subsequently, she slammed open the counselor's door and proceeded at a rapid pace to leave the school with the counselor and psychologist in pursuit. The counselor and consultant simply had to ride out the storm. Afterwards she was most remorseful. Since this was not the first incident and because she was a suicidal risk, she also was hospitalized that afternoon.

When considering the severity of the agitation, both the frequency and intensity of the excessive behavior and temper outbursts are considered. Agitation is considered to be symptomatic when the child is frequently unable to sit still and/or is frequently disruptive because of either excessive behavior or angry outbursts.

MULTIPLE MANIFESTATIONS OF DEPRESSION

From the preceding discussion, it is apparent that each symptom of the depressive disorder is destructive by itself. The simultaneous occurrence of multiple symptoms compounds the debilitating impact of each symptom. For a child to receive a diagnosis of depression, multiple symptoms must be present. In the case of major depression, five symptoms must be present at the same time. Similarly, three symptoms must be present at the same time for a diagnosis of dysthymic disorder. However, these figures represent the minimum number of symptoms that must be present for a diagnosis. The child may exhibit many more symptoms. In fact, researchers suggest (Brumback et al., 1977) that 50% of depressed children experience seven or more symptoms. The author's own research indicates that the child from a public school who is experiencing major depression reports having an average of eight clinically relevant symptoms and quite a few additional symptoms that are experienced at a more moderate level.

DIAGNOSIS OF DEPRESSION IN CHILDREN

In the preceding sections of this chapter, the variety of symptoms that are associated with the syndrome of depression were described. However, not all of these symptoms enter into the equation when one is making a diagnosis of a depressive disorder according to the DSM-III-R (APA, 1987). The symptoms and other manifestations of childhood depression that are not considered when one is making a diagnostic decision are referred to as "associated features," and they will be discussed in a subsequent section of this chapter. In this section of the chapter, the diagnostic criteria for the depressive disorders will be discussed. The mood disorders characterized by a manic episode either in isolation or in combination with a depressive episode will not be considered in this chapter. The interested reader is directed to DSM-III-R as well as relevant review articles (cf. Strober & Carlson, 1982).

There are three primary diagnostic categories of depressive disorders, including major depression, dysthymic disorder, and depressive disorder not otherwise specified. All three disorders are characterized by a primary disturbance of depressed mood accompanied by other symptoms that clearly are not a result of another physical or mental disorder. The primary difference between the three disorders is the number, severity, and duration of depressive symptoms.

Major Depression

The syndrome of major depression in children is characterized by a prominent and persistent symptom of dysphoric mood or anhedonia. In addition to the mood disorder, the syndrome also includes at least four of the following symptoms: (1) eating disturbance and unusual weight gain or loss; (2) sleep disturbance; (3) psychomotor retardation or agitation; (4) anhedonia or diminished interest in usual activities; (5) fatigue; (6) negative self-evaluations or excessive guilt; (7) difficulty concentrating; and (8) recurrent thoughts of death, suicidal ideation, or suicidal behavior. For a diagnosis of major depression, four or more of these symptoms must be present nearly every day over a period of at least 2 weeks.

A number of exclusionary criteria that preclude a diagnosis of major depression also are delineated in DSM-III-R. Such a diagnosis would be inappropriate if the child is experiencing mood-incongruent delusions or hallucinations or bizarre behavior. In addition, if the child exhibits schizophrenia, schizophreniform disorder, or a paranoid disorder prior to or during the depressive episode, it precludes a diagnosis of major depression. Similarly, if an organic mental disorder or an uncomplicated bereavement is evident, a diagnosis of major depression would be inappropriate.

Dysthymic Disorder

Dysthymic disorder, sometimes referred to as either minor or neurotic depression, is similar in nature to major depression, but the symptoms are less severe and may be shorter in duration. Dysthymic disorder is characterized by a chronic mood disturbance of either dysphoria or anger and a number of other symptoms associated with a depressive disorder. The symptoms must be present for a minimum of 1 year's duration. However, the symptoms may be separated by periods of normality a couple of weeks in duration but no longer than a few months at a time.

During the periods of mood disturbance, at least two of the following symptoms must also be present: (1) sleep disturbance; (2) fatigue; (3) negative self-evaluations; (4) decreased academic performance; (5) decreased concentration; (6) social withdrawal; (7) anhedonia; (8) irritability or anger expressed toward caretakers; (9) inability to respond with pleasure to praise or rewards; (10) moderate levels of psychomotor retardation; (11) hopelessness or self-pity; (12) excessive weepiness; (13) recurrent thoughts of death or suicide. A diagnosis of dysthymic disorder would be precluded by the presence of psychotic features such as bizarre behavior or a thought disturbance.

Depressive Disorder Not Otherwise Specified

Children who exhibit depressive symptoms but do not meet the diagnostic criteria for either major depression or dysthymic disorder and do not exhibit any manic behavior may receive a diagnosis of depressive disorder not otherwise specified. Such a diagnosis would be given in the case of the child who exhibits the symptomatology of dysthymic disorder but whose symptom-free periods last longer than a few months. Other examples would include a youngster who has a chronic low-grade sadness or a child who has schizophrenia, residual type, that develops without psychotic features but also includes a distinct and sustained episode of major depression.

DEPRESSION AND
SPECIAL EDUCATION CLASSIFICATION

Even though a child may receive a DSM-III-R diagnosis of depression, according to federal regulations the child may not qualify for special education placement. For a child to qualify for special education services, the child must have a problem that is adversely affecting his or her performance in school. As noted in Chapter 2, the academic performance of depressed youths is significantly lower than that for nondepressed children. However, a closer look at the results of one of the author's studies (Stark, Livingston, Laurent, & Cardenas, 1990), indicates that these youngsters were still passing at an average to above-average level. Thus, the decrement in performance may not be so severe that it leads to failure, nor may it qualify as an "educational need." Thus, it is especially important when evaluating the educational programming needs of a depressed child to compare how the child is functioning scholastically and socially at the present time to how the child was functioning in those same two areas prior to the depressive episode. This difference often is great enough to document an educational need.

In the cases where an educational need can be documented, the depressed child could qualify for special education under the classification of severely emotionally disturbed. If such a classification is being pursued, then two additional general criteria must be met for the child to qualify. The disturbance must be evident to a marked degree, and it must have existed for a relatively long time. If the three aforementioned criteria are met, then the child must exhibit one of the five disturbances identified in the federal regulations. The depressed youth would qualify under the fourth of these disturbances: the child exhibits a severe and pervasive depressed mood.

Similar to considering the ramifications of special education placement for any child, there are a number of things that must be given greater consideration when one makes such a programming decision for a depressed youth. Foremost among these is how the youth will perceive the move. What will it mean to the child about him- or herself to be in special education? Since depressed children have a negative sense of self, such a move could confirm in their own mind that they are deficient. Thus, care must be taken when discussing the placement with the child. Furthermore, the psychologist must put him- or herself into the child's shoes and try to determine how the child will perceive the new environment. "I must be a bad kid, I'm in with all of the troublemakers." "I'm a loser, why else would I be with the dirtballs." "I always knew that I'm stupid." Then, the perception that is likely to be created must be dealt with and reframed or disputed using the techniques noted in Chapter 4. Alternatively, if the child's negative interpretation is based to a significant extent on reality (the depressed child is being placed in a class of delinquents), then special education placement may need to be reconsidered.

Will the special education placement foster independence or breed dependence? Since depressed children often are regressive, the youngster may become dependent on the resource teacher for academic and emotional support. This may be appropriate at first, but the programming must have built into it steps that will lead to independence.

Will special education placement exacerbate the child's problems with social withdrawal? Will the child lose contact with his or her good friends? A lot of this impact will depend on the extent of resource programming versus mainstreaming. Thus, it is important to ensure that the special education placement does not lead to further social isolation.

Is the special education curriculum appropriate for the child? Commonly the portion of the programming that is designed to foster an improved sense of self is helpful. However, the oftentimes punitive behavior management systems are countertherapeutic. A positive system that emphasizes rewards for appropriate behavior and accomplishments is necessary. In a related vein, will the resource room provide the child with the extra support he or she needs to improve his or her schoolwork? It is important that the child receives help during study time and that he or she is not allowed to spend that time napping.

Finally, it is critical for the special education teacher and psychologist to be continually vigilant for the child's negative thoughts surrounding the special educational programming and its meaning for the child about him- or herself. Distortions in thinking should be restructured using the procedures described in Chapter 4.

ASSOCIATED FEATURES

As noted in the introduction to this chapter, there are a number of maladaptive emotions, behaviors, and thoughts that commonly co-occur with the symptoms that are evaluated when one makes a diagnosis of a depressive disorder. They are referred to as "associated features" in DSM-III-R. A number of these associated features are specific to depressed adults, whereas others are evident across the life span. Still others are specific to children and adolescents, and they are referred to as "age-specific associated features."

Non-Age-Specific Associated Features

The associated features that we have found to be relevant to children are behaviors and emotions such as depressed appearance, excessive weepiness, feelings of anxiety, irritability, brooding, excessive concern with physical health, and phobias. Two of these features, excessive weepiness and irritability, have already been described and consequently will be excluded from the following discussion.

Depressed Appearance

Many of the depressed children we have interviewed looked sad. Their lips were down-turned, they gave a minimum of eye contact, on occasion their tear ducts would well up, and they rarely smiled. Other children were simply devoid of emotion. Although these clinical impressions regarding the nonverbal behavior of depressed children are consistent with what one would expect given a knowledge of depressive symptomatology, researchers (Kazdin, Esveldt-Dawson, Sherick, & Colbus, 1985) have not been able empirically to differentiate depressed from nondepressed children. We recently completed a study in which depressed and nondepressed children were video-taped in a free-interaction situation. Using a more microscopic analysis of nonverbal social behavior, we anticipate being able to isolate empirically some of the variables that differentiate the children. Preliminary results are promising.

Excess Anxiety

Children who are depressed also report significantly higher than normal levels of anxiety (Stark, Laurent, Rouse, & Printz, 1990). In fact, anxiety disorders may be the most common disorders that occur simultaneously with an episode of depression (Kovacs, 1985). In a recently completed study (Laurent, 1989), the prevalence of coexisting anxiety disorders was investigated. Half of the depressed children had at least one concurrent anxiety disorder, and 14% of the depressed youngsters had two anxiety disorders concurrent with an episode of depression. The most common coexisting anxiety disorder was overanxious disorder, which was the anxiety disorder that was diagnosed among half of the depressed and anxious children. Separation anxiety was the next most commonly diagnosed coexisting anxiety disorder. It was reported by 20% of the depressed youngsters, and, when there were multiple anxiety disorders present, separation anxiety was one of them. A less severe anxiety disorder that is referred to as "anxiety disorder not otherwise specified" was identified among 13% of the depressed children. Finally, 13% of the depressed children reported a simple phobia.

The extent of the relationship between the syndromes of depression and anxiety is unclear at this time because of the methodological limitations of existing research. Previous research relied solely on self-report instruments to assess the presence and severity of depression and anxiety. In Chapter 3 it will become apparent that this approach is fraught with limitations. A recently published study (Wolfe et al., 1987) raises questions about the validity of the commonly used self-report measures of depression and anxiety in children. Thus, it appears as though it is important for future investigators to assess the presence and severity of both depressive and anxious symptomatology using a semistructured interview such as the K-SADS.

Health Concerns

Some depressed children exhibit excessive concern about their health. They may even obsess about it. The slightest bodily reaction is interpreted as a sign of a physical malady. For example, a stomachache may be interpreted as the beginning of an ulcer or of the stomach rotting out. This concern may even prevent affected children from engaging in recreational activities. They do not believe that their bodies can handle it. They complain to their teachers about feeling sick and consequently spend a great deal of time in the nurse's office. In addition, they have paid significantly more visits to doctors' offices than their peers. The children can recite a lengthy history of physical concerns such as rotting organs that the physicians they visited could not diagnose or treat.

Phobias

Some depressed children also report phobias. Perhaps the most common phobia among children that is also associated with depression is school phobia. Some form of school refusal was found in 62% of Brumback et al.'s (1977) sample of depressed youths. The school-phobic child experiences an intense fear of school. The child may refuse to leave the house to go to school. He or she may physically resist leaving the home. For example, a child may grab onto the door to prevent someone from removing him from the house. Likewise, the child might wedge his or her legs on either side of a car door to prevent him- or herself from being removed from the car.

Age-Specific Associated Features

In DSM-III-R, one age-specific associated feature is noted for depressed children. It is separation anxiety. We have not identified any depressed fourth- through sixth-grade children who were experiencing separation anxiety. However, in an earlier investigation (Reynolds, Wysopal, & Stark, 1984), we did identify a depressed third grader who was also experiencing separation anxiety. She described it in the following way. When asked if she thought about death, she burst into tears. After taking some time to collect herself, she reported that she thought a lot about her parents dying. Every day she was afraid that they would be killed on the way to or from work. If they were late getting home, she would become petrified that they had been killed on the highway. Illness of a parent also was traumatic. She had difficulty paying attention to her teachers because she was thinking about her parents dying. In other cases, fear of separation may be so intense that the child refuses to go to school. A number of other investigators have also reported an association between depression in children and separation anxiety (Puig-Antich, Blau, Marx, Greenhill, & Chambers, 1978).

Additional age-specific associated features have been reported for depressed adolescents. These features have been found among our fourth- through sixth-grade samples. A number of these features were described above including irritability and anger, social with-

drawal, diminished school performance, agitation, and feeling unloved. A few additional features were noted in DSM-III-R and will
be described below.

Running Away

Running away from home is an expression of the depressed youngster's attempts to withdraw from the problems that are seen as insur-
mountable. Running away seems to be most prevalent among depressed girls. Depressed youths tend to run away more frequently
than their nondepressed peers, and the precipitating events may be
less severe than the ones that cause a nondepressed youth to run
away. We treat an attempt to run away in a similar manner to a
suicide attempt. It is viewed as a message that the child is experiencing an intolerable level of stress.

Feeling Misunderstood

Many adolescents feel misunderstood by their parents and other
authority figures. This feeling appears to be exacerbated when the
youngster is also experiencing an episode of depression. Such youngsters believe that no one understands them. These feelings are especially strong after a reprimand or any other indication that they have
done something wrong. These youngsters act as though they have a
"chip on their shoulders." They may snap "you don't understand" and
then walk away in anger.

Other Noticeable Changes

Depressed adolescents may exhibit a number of other unusual behaviors around the house. The youth may be uncooperative with his
or her parents and respond with belligerence or withdrawal. The
parents might notice that their son or daughter is sulking more than
usual or seems exceptionally emotional. Finally, the youngster may
be paying less attention to his or her appearance.

NATURAL COURSE OF DEPRESSION
DURING CHILDHOOD

As noted in the introduction to this chapter, depression is a syndrome that is comprised of a number of symptoms that reliably co-

occur. Through the description of the symptoms that comprise the syndrome, it may have become apparent that depression is a very serious disorder that has a broad impact on a child's life. When one considers the gravity of the disruption in a child's life that results from an episode of depression, it would seem as though the length of the episode may, in part, mediate both the short- and long-term impact of the syndrome on the child's psychosocial well-being. The longer the duration of the episode, the more pervasive the impact. Evidence suggests that episodes of depression are both long-lasting and recurrent.

Kovacs and colleagues (Kovacs, Feinberg, Crouse-Novak, Paulas-kos, & Finkelstein, 1984; Kovacs, Feinberg, Crouse-Novak, Pau-laskos, Pollock, et al., 1984b) have conducted a 5-year longitudinal study of depression among children. They found the average length of an episode of major depression to be 7½ months and the average length of an episode of dysthymic disorder to be 3 years. The natural recovery rate for an episode of the two disorders also is different and, in the case of dysthymic disorder, quite protracted. Approximately 92% of the children with major depression recovered from the episode within a year and a half. On the other hand, after 6½ years, 89% of the children with dysthymic disorder recovered from their current episode. In both cases, the younger the age at first onset, the longer the period of recovery. Furthermore, children with either disorder are at high risk for a later episode. Children who had major depression stood a 72% chance of another episode within 5 years. Moreover, the periods of normality between episodes were found to be relatively short: not in excess of 2 years. Children who were suffering from dysthymic disorders were at high risk for one or a few concurrent episode(s) of major depression.

A number of other investigators have completed research of a less systematic nature that addresses the natural course of depression in children. Brumback et al. (1977) reported that the average length of an episode of depression was 20 weeks. Puig-Antich (1982) noted that the average length of a depressive episode was 1 to 2 years. Geller, Chestnut, Miller, Price, and Yates (1985) found the episodes of depression among children to be much longer than those reported in the two aforementioned studies. Geller and colleagues noted that 86% of their sample had depressive episodes that were longer than 2 years in duration, and nearly 56% had episodes lasting over 5 years. Poznanski, Krahenbuhl, and Zrull (1976) reported similar results. Of the 10 depressed youths they reassessed 6½ years later, 50% still were depressed.

DEMOGRAPHIC CHARACTERISTICS OF
DEPRESSED YOUTHS

A summary of the demographic characteristics of the depressed youngsters identified through the first 3 years of the author's research is reported in Table 1.2. An interesting finding, and one that is found quite consistently, is that it appears as through the number of depressed boys is similar to the number of depressed girls. This is quite unlike the depressed adult population, where the number of depressed females is reported to be twice as great as the number of depressed males. Thus, our research would suggest that this gender difference must appear later, perhaps during adolescence. At the present time, there is an accumulating body of evidence that suggests that the depressed boys in our sample of school children are more severely impaired than the girls. The boys' profiles in a number of studies have been more like those found among severely depressed adults, whereas the girls' results have been more characteris-

TABLE 1.2. Demographic Information on the Total Sample of Depressed School Children (*n* = 61)

Gender	
Boys	45%
Girls	55%
Race	
Anglo	82.5%
Hispanic	12.5%
Black	5%
Educational program	
Regular	95%
Learning disabilities	5%
Living arrangement	
Biological parents	45%
Mother	15%
Mother and stepfather	27.5%
Father and stepmother	2.5%
Father	7.5%
Other	2.5%

Note. Information on the grades the children were in was not included because the data would have been misleading. A disproportionately high number of sixth graders have participated in the research project, and a disproportionately low number of seventh graders have participated in the research.

tic of mild to moderately depressed adults. These results have occurred even though there is no difference between girls and boys in
regard to their severity ratings on the K-SADS or CDI.

The racial composition of the depressed sample was quite consistent with the racial composition of the larger sample from which it
was drawn. The majority of the youngsters (82.5%) were white,
12.5% were Hispanic, and 5% were black. Previous research (cf.
Kovacs, Feinburg, Crouse-Novak, Paulaskos, & Finkelstein, 1984)
indicated that depression is more common among children from
lower-SES families. The author's research group has not systematically collected data on this topic. However, some informal findings
suggest that this may be true among the school children. First, a
disproportionate number of the depressed youths have lived in the
areas of the community that have a high concentration of mobile
homes, apartment complexes, and duplexes. Thus, if the cost of
their housing is an accurate reflection of family income, it would
appear as though more of the depressed youngsters are coming from
lower-SES families. Another possible predictor of family income is
marital status. The family income in single-parent households tends
to be lower than that for two-parent families. Twenty-two percent of
the depressed youths came from single-parent families.

The vast majority of the depressed children (95%) were enrolled
in the regular education program. These youngsters' special needs
had not been identified by school personnel. This may not be surprising, since these children are generally well-behaved, quiet, and
sensitive students who are not annoying their teachers. Consequently, they are not referred for special education services.

Fewer than half (45%) of the depressed children were living with both
of their biological parents. Fifty-five percent were from broken homes,
with 22.5% living in single-parent families, 30% living in stepfamilies,
and another 2.5% living with other relatives. There are a myriad of
possible reasons why there would be a disproportionately high number
of depressed children from broken homes. As noted earlier, there are
financial hardships associated with a divorce that could lead to greater
stress. The youngster may be reacting to the loss of a significant other.
Perhaps one or both of the parents were psychologically disturbed,
which led to the divorce. Another possibility is that the bickering and
bad feelings that preceded the dissolution of the family contributed to
the child's problems. The list of possibilities is enormous, and it is very
likely that there are multiple contributing factors rather than a single
causal factor. From a practical standpoint, it will take some astute
clinical work to wade through the myriad of possible contributing factors to identify the most salient ones for each child.

2

Review of Relevant Research on Prevalence, Family Interactions, and Treatments

This chapter focuses on research that establishes the scope of the problem of depression among children as well as implications for how to treat depressed youths. Included are a review of epidemiological studies and investigations of the impact of depression on the intellectual and academic functioning of depressed children. Since the depressed youngster's family can play a critical role in the development, maintenance, and treatment of depression, research into the interactions of families with a depressed child will be discussed. Finally, the existing treatment outcome literature will be reviewed. From this review, it will become apparent that there is a very limited empirical knowledge base about childhood depression. However, existing evidence indicates that depression affects a relatively large number of school-aged children, and it impacts on both the child's psychosocial and intellectual/academic functioning.

PREVALENCE OF DEPRESSION AMONG CHILDREN

For many reasons the prevalence of depression among children has been underestimated for years. Within the professional community, there was debate about its very existence, and, were the phenomenon to exist, its clinical picture. Within our culture, it is commonly believed that childhood is a carefree, happy time. Surely there could not be any reason for a child to be depressed. Because of the highly subjective nature of depression, it often goes unnoticed by parents and school personnel. There is, in fact, evidence that indicates that depression is underdiagnosed by referral sources such as parents, school personnel, and family physicians. The vast majority of the depressed children the author's research group has identified through the assessment procedure described in Chapter 3 had gone unnoticed by school personnel and parents. This is not surprising, since they do not command attention. They commonly are the quiet, well-behaved, and sensitive children who try to please adults. It is the rowdy, acting-out, disciplinary problem who commands the most attention and energy from school personnel.

When some of the symptoms of depression are noticed by an adult, it often is assumed that the child is going through a "phase" that he or she will outgrow. A number of parents have stated that they just thought their child was lazy and had derided him or her for this character flaw. This led to hard feelings on the part of all involved, and the child experienced a sense of rejection. Certainly, this does not have a positive impact on the youngster's self-esteem.

What is the actual prevalence of depression among children? It appears as though there is not a simple answer to this question. The prevalence varies widely across investigations (see Table 2.1) for a variety of reasons that are listed in Table 2.2. First, the prevalence appears to vary according to the population being studied (Carlson & Cantwell, 1979). There is a lower rate found among children in the general population relative to at-risk populations such as offspring of depressed parents and children with life-threatening diseases, and the highest rates are found among children who comprise psychiatric populations.

Different diagnostic criteria have been utilized across investigations (Cantwell, 1983), which has contributed to the differences in prevalence reported by investigators. Since 1980, most investigators have used DSM-III criteria. However, prior to 1980, investigators used their own criteria (see Weinberg, Rutman, Sullivan, Penick, & Dietz, 1973), and in other studies it is unclear what criteria were used (see Carlson & Cantwell, 1980). With the advent of DSM-III-R, there was a small change in the diagnostic criteria for dysthymic disorder. To make a diagnosis of dysthymic disorder using DSM-III criteria, among other things the youngster had to exhibit dysphoric mood plus three additional symptoms. In contrast, using DSM-III-R, the same diagnosis can be made for a child who exhibits dysphoric mood plus two additional symptoms. Thus, with the less stringent criteria, it is possible that more children would receive such a diagnosis.

The method employed for identifying depressed children also varied across studies. Some investigators relied solely on self-report measures to identify depressed youths (see Albert & Beck, 1975), whereas others interviewed an entire sample of children (e.g., Pfeffer et al., 1984). Other investigators have used a multiple-gate assessment procedure where children were first screened with a paper-and-pencil measure, and then those children who scored above a given cut-off score were interviewed (e.g., Kashani et al., 1983). Still others retrospectively reviewed case notes in clients' folders as a means of identifying depressed subjects (e.g., Poznanski & Zrull, 1970).

A few investigators used a single source of information such as the child (Albert & Beck, 1975) for making diagnostic decisions, whereas most investigators combined information from the child and a parent to make a diagnosis. Others combined multiple sources of information such as child, parent, hospital staff, and other professionals who knew the child (e.g., Kashani, Lababidi, & Jones, 1982). Lefkowitz and Tesiny (1985) relied on peers to identify depressed youngsters. The prevalence of depression appears to vary according to who the informant was (Lobovits & Handal, 1985).

The age of the children studied varied across investigations, which contributes to differences in prevalence rates (Kazdin, French, Unis, Esveldt-Dawson, & Sherick, 1983). The rate appears to increase with age. Children as young as preschool age have been studied (Frommer, Mendelson, & Reid, 1972), whereas other investigators have included youths who were 17 years old in their samples (Kashani & Hakami, 1982). In the majority of investigations, adolescents were mixed in with children as young as 6 and 7 years.

A methodological concern that has been overlooked at times is the establishment of interrater reliability for the diagnoses. Thus, in such cases the degree of agreement in diagnoses is unknown, which in fact may contribute to differences in prevalence rates (Lobovits & Handal, 1985). In a somewhat related vein, Lobovits and Handal have noted that the stringency of the diagnostic criteria used for determining whether a youngster was depressed varied across studies—the more stringent the criteria, the lower the prevalence rate (Carlson & Cantwell, 1980).

In most of the investigations reported in Table 2.1, the authors only reported the occurrence of major depression. Since this was the only diagnostic criterion reported in the methods section, it is assumed that the investigators did not identify children who were exhibiting dysthymic disorder or depressive disorder not otherwise specified. It would seem logical that the fewer the possible depressive disorders included in the study, the lower the prevalence rate, and the more possible disorders included in the study, the higher the prevalence rate. The investigation conducted by Kashani et al.

TABLE 2.1. Incidence of Depression across Populations of Children

Authors	Population	*n*	Age in years	Racial composition[a]	Sex
Lefkowitz & Tesiny, 1985	General school	3,020	$\overline{X}=9.83$	50.6% W 30.5% B 6.2% H 2.9% O	51% M
Kashani & Simonds, 1979	General	103	7–12	NA	49% M
Kashani, Barbero, et al., 1981	General New Zealand	100	9	NA	NA
Pfeffer et al., 1984	General school	101	6–12	75% W 25% O	70% M
	Inpatients	65	6–12	75% W 25% O	70% M
Albert & Beck, 1975	General school	63	11–15	98% W 2% O	54% M
Weinberg et al., 1973	Educational diagnostic clinic	72	6.5–12.75	100% W	69% M
Lobovits & Handal, 1985	Academic and/or behavioral problems	50	8–12	NA	74% M
Ling et al., 1970	Headache patients	25	4–16	100% W	50% M
Kashani, Barbero, et al., 1981	General medical patients	100	7–12	88% W 9% B 2% O 2% I	56% M
Kashani, Venzke, et al., 1981	Orthopedic patients	100	7–12	NA	48% M
Kashani & Hakani, 1982	Cancer patients	35	6–17	97% W 3% O	71% M

Assessment instrumentations	Sources of information	Diagnostic criteria	Results
PNID, modified CDI	Peers	None	5.2% Severe depressive symptomatology
Interview	Mother and child	DSM-III	1.9% Major 17.4% Sadness with additional symptoms

Screening measure followed by K-SADS interview	Child and parent	DSM-III	Current:
			  1.8% Major
			  2.5% Dysthymic
			Past:
			  1.1% Major
			  9.7% Dysthymic
			Current:
			  2.4% Major
			  4.4% Dysthymic
			Past:
			  2.0% Major
			  7.2% Dysthymic

Interview	Mother and child	DSM-III	0% Major 13.9% Dysthymic
Interview	Mother and child	DSM-III	20% Major 13.8% Dysthymic
BDI	Child	None	33.3% Moderate 2.2% Severe
Interview	Parent and child	Authors'	49% Currently 10% Previously
Interview, CDI, PIC-D	Child and mother	DSM-III	34% Child report 22% Parent report
Review files and interview	Multiple	Authors'	40% Depressed
Interview, BDI, other	Child, mother, and other	DSM-III	7% Major
Interview	Child and parents	DSM-III	23% Major
Interview and other	Child, mother, and other	DSM-III	17% Major

(continued)

TABLE 2.1. (cont.)

Authors	Population	n	Age in years	Racial composition[a]	Sex
Kashani et al., 1985	Children of mood-disordered parents	50	7–17	88% W 12% B	54% M
Poznanski & Zrull, 1970	Outpatients	66	7–12 0–6	NA NA	NA NA
Colbert et al., 1982	Inpatients	282	6–14	NA	NA
Frommer et al., 1972	Inpatients	210	0–5	NA	59% M
Kashani et al., 1982	Inpatients	100	NA	NA	NA
Christ et al., 1981	Inpatients	10,412	6–16	50% W 50% B	64.5% M
Petti, 1978	Inpatients	73	6–12.5	NA	NA
Carlson & Cantwell, 1980	In- and outpatients	210	7–17	70% W	65% M

[a]W=white; B=black; H=Hispanic; I=American Indian; and O=other.

(1983) is a good example of this. When major depression is looked at in isolation, the prevalence rate is 1.8%. However, when both major depression and dysthymic disorder are considered together, the prevalence rate is 4.3%. Thus, the rate more than doubles. If Pfeffer et al. (1984) had solely identified children with major depression in their normal school population, they would have reported that depression was nonexistent in the school population. In stark contrast to this, they reported that almost 14% of their sample reported a dysthymic disorder.

A final consideration when trying to understand the myriad of prevalence rates of depression among children is whether the investigators reported the current rate of depression or the lifetime rate. In the former case, only the number of children who were depressed at the time of the study go into the formula when computing the prevalence. In the latter case, the number of children who were depressed at any previous time and those who are currently depressed are combined and entered into the equation to compute prevalence

Assessment instrumentations	Sources of information	Diagnostic criteria	Results
Interview	Child and mother	DSM-III	Child report: Unipolar parent 13% Bipolar parent 22% Parent report: Unipolar parent 2% Bipolar parent 12%
Case records Case records	Case records, multiple sources	NA	15% 12.5%
NA	NA	DSM-III	54%
Records	Review records	Authors'	58% Depressive symptomatology
Interview and other	Child, mother, and other professionals	DSM-III	15% Major
Records	Multiple	DSM-I or -II	2.1% Psychotic 11.7% Neurotic
Interview and other	Child, parent, and other	Weinberg criteria	61%
Interview	Child	NA	25% Depressive

rates. Obviously, the lifetime rate is higher. For example, Kashani et al. (1983) reported that 4.3% of the children were currently depressed and another 10.8% were depressed in the past, producing a lifetime rate of 15.1%.

General Population

The prevalence of depression among the general school population of children ranges from 1.9% (Kashani & Simonds, 1979) to 13.9% (Pfeffer et al., 1984). On the low end, Kashani and Simonds reported that 1.9% of their sample of children were experiencing major depression. This figure is similar to the 1.8% Kashani and colleagues found in 1983 and is greater than the 0% reported by Pfeffer et al. Kashani et al. (1983) report a second figure in their study of 2.4% for major depression. This stems from the fact that they used a screening device to identify children whom they subsequently interviewed. This procedure yielded the 1.8% rating. However, a validity

TABLE 2.2. Reasons for Differences in Prevalence Rates of Depression among Children

---

1. Different populations were studied.
2. Different diagnostic criteria were utilized.
3. Different methods were used to identify children who were depressed.
4. The informant utilized for assessing depression varied.
5. Different measures were used for quantifying the presence and severity of depressive symptomatology.
6. Different ages of children were studied.
7. In some investigations there was a failure to compute interrater reliability for diagnoses.
8. The degree of stringency required for a diagnosis varied.
9. Some investigations only report the prevalence of major depression, whereas others include dysthymic, bipolar, and cyclothymic disorders.
10. Current rates are reported in some studies, whereas other investigators report lifetime rates.

---

check of their procedure revealed that their screening device under-identified children as depressed. In a second sample of children that was not subject to this limitation, they found a prevalence rate of 2.4%. In our own research in the schools (Stark, Laurent, Rouse, & Printz, 1990), using a multiple-gate assessment procedure (see Chapter 3), we have found a prevalence rate for major depression of 1%.

Dysthymic disorder appears to be more prevalent than major depression among the general school population. Kashani et al. (1983) reported current prevalence rates of 2.5% and 4.4%, whereas Pfeffer et al. (1984) reported a current rate of 13.9%. When lifetime rates are computed, Kashani et al. reported rates of 2.9% and 4.4% for major depression and 12.2% for dysthymic disorder. Once again, our own research (e.g., Stark, Laurent, et al., 1990) over a 3-year period indicates that about 1% of the general school population report a current diagnosable dysthymic disorder. However, unlike previous investigators, we also kept track of the number of children who were diagnosed as depressive disorder not otherwise specified. These children reported a long-standing experience of dysphoria, low self-esteem, and two additional symptoms. We found a prevalence rate of 2.6% for this disorder. Thus, when all three diagnostic groups were considered simultaneously, a prevalence figure of approximately 4% was found.

In two other investigations, the authors did not interview their subjects and thus could not make formal diagnoses. Instead, they used paper-and-pencil measures that had cut-off scores that indicated severe levels of depressive symptomatology. Lefkowitz and Tesiny (1985) used a Peer Nomination Inventory of Depression (PNID) to identify depressed youths. This instrument identified 5.2% of their sample as exhibiting severe levels of depressive symptomatology. This rate is close to the 4.3% reported by Kashani et al. (1983) but less than their second figure of 6.8% and less than half of Pfeffer's 13.9%. In the other investigation that used a paper-and-pencil measure, Albert and Beck studied an early adolescent population that completed a modified version of the Beck Depression Inventory (BDI; Beck, Ward, Mendelson, Mock, & Erlbough, 1961). They found that 33.3% of their sample reported a moderate level of depressive symptomatology when using adult cut-off scores. This figure seems unreasonably high. They also found that 2.2% of the youngsters reported a severe level of depressive symptomatology. This latter figure is more in line with other research.

Special Populations

Perhaps the studies from this genre that are of greatest relevance to school psychologists are those that involve children with educational difficulties. Evidence and common sense would suggest that children who were having academic or behavioral difficulties would be at risk for emotional problems. The difficulties the children experience at school negatively impact their self-esteem, and low self-esteem is one of the cardinal symptoms of depression.

Weinberg et al. (1973) interviewed children who were referred to an educational diagnostic clinic and their parents. Results indicated that 49% of the children were depressed at the time of the interview, and another 10% had been depressed in the past. Lobovits and Handal (1985) assessed depression among children referred to a psychiatric clinic for behavioral and academic problems. Their results were somewhat lower. According to self-report information, 34% of the youngsters were depressed. On the basis of information from the children's mothers, 22% of the children were depressed. Both of these rates were lower than those reported above by Weinberg and colleagues. This may be a reflection of the fact that the Weinberg sample was more homogeneous and consisted of more children with educational difficulties and fewer with behavioral problems.

Children with a variety of medical problems face extreme, and in some cases chronic, stress, which may place them at risk for depression (Best & Stark, 1990). Researchers have found relatively elevated levels of depression among children presenting with headaches

(40%; Ling, Oftedal, & Weinberg, 1970), general medical patients (7%; Kashani, Venzke, & Miller, 1981), orthopedic patients (23%; Kashani, Venzke, et al., 1981), and cancer patients (17%; Kashani & Hakami, 1982). The previously noted figures, with the exception of the Ling study, are for children who have been given a DSM-III diagnosis of major depression. In the Ling et al. study, the author's own diagnostic criteria were used, although their criteria were very similar to those required for a DSM-II diagnosis of major depression. It may be that all of the aforementioned figures are an underestimate, since the investigators did not identify children with dysthymic disorder or depressive disorder not otherwise specified. The relatively high rate found in the Ling study may be a reflection of the fact that these youngsters presented with a subjective somatic complaint (headache). One of the most frequent symptoms of depression is somatic complaints, of which headaches are one of the more common complaints. In the case of the medical patients, it appears as though the degree of severity and life change posed by the type of problem may be a determinant of the frequency of depression in the population. In the case of the cancer patients, death was a real concern, and the patients were faced with prolonged, painful treatment procedures that caused noticeable changes in their appearance. Likewise, most of the orthopedic patients were facing either surgery or physical therapy. Many of these patients had noticeable handicaps that limited their social activities.

A final at-risk population is children of depressed parents. Kashani, Burk, and Reid (1985) reported that 13% of children of unipolar depressed parents are depressed according to self-report information, and 22% of the children of bipolar depressed parents were depressed.

Psychiatric Patients

A wide age range of inpatient and outpatient samples have been studied to determine the prevalence of depression among psychiatric patients. Depression is considered to be rare among preschool-age children (Kashani & Ray, 1985). However, results of two studies suggest that it may not be as rare among preschool-age psychiatric patients. Poznanski and Zrull (1970) reported that 12.5% of their sample of outpatient children were depressed. Frommer et al. (1972) did not formally diagnose their preschool sample, but they did assess for depressive symptomatology. A large percentage of these youngsters (58%) exhibited depressive symptomatology. It is important to recognize that the symptoms of depression are fairly common and that depressive disorders are much less common (Carlson & Cantwell, 1982).

The prevalence of depression among elementary-age children involved in psychiatric treatment ranges from 2.1% to 61%. On the low end, Christ, Adler, Isacoff, and Gershansky (1981) reviewed 1,042 case files and found that 2.1% could be diagnosed as psychotically depressed using DSM-I and DSM-II criteria. Another 11.7% were diagnosed as being neurotically depressed. The combined rate is fairly consistent with the 15% reported by Poznanski and Zrull (1970) and the 13% reported by Kashani et al. (1982). In this latter study, the authors only reported the prevalence of major depression. Perhaps this is a reflection of the fact that they treat dysthymic disordered youths as outpatients, and they studied an inpatient population. Carlson and Cantwell (1980) reported a somewhat higher figure of 25% for a combined group of inpatients and outpatients. Since they did not designate the diagnoses of the children, it is not possible to determine whether this higher figure results from the authors including children who were diagnosed with either major depression or dysthymic disorder.

In two investigations the authors reported relatively high prevalence rates. Colbert, Newman, Ney, and Young (1982) reported that 54% of their inpatient sample of 6- to 14-year-olds were depressed according to DSM-III criteria. However, the types of disorders were not stated, and their procedure was unclear. Petti (1978) used a very sound procedure of interviewing the children, their parents, and other sources of information to derive diagnoses, and he reported a prevalence rate of 61% using Weinberg's (Weinberg et al., 1973) criteria. Research indicates that Weinberg and DSM-III criteria for major depression are comparable. Thus, the difference in diagnostic criteria used by the investigators can be ruled out as an explanation for the differences. Regardless, results across the aforementioned studies suggest that depressed children comprise a relatively large proportion of the children referred to psychiatric clinics.

INTELLECTUAL IMPAIRMENT AND DEPRESSION IN CHILDREN

A number of the symptoms of depression are likely to have an adverse impact on the academic performance of a youngster. Specifically, anhedonia, negative self-evaluations, difficulty concentrating, indecisiveness, fatigue, and psychomotor retardation or agitation could lead to a failure to perform academic tasks at a level commensurate with one's ability and predepression level. Some of the symptoms affect the child's motivation, whereas others affect the efficiency of the youngster's cognitive processing. As noted in Chapter 1, the anhedonic individual does not derive or experience pleasure from the usual experiences. Such an individual does not experience the sense of satisfaction associated with successful learning experiences and, consequently, loses a source of reinforcement and motivation for learning. The youngster who negatively evaluates his or her performance also is likely to be less motivated in school, since he or she is not going to attain a level of performance that is commensurate with his or her standards. Rather, the child repeatedly will castigate him- or herself for perceived inadequacies and failures.

Obviously, the child who is having trouble concentrating is going to have difficulties focusing on the information presented in class, which limits the acquisition of knowledge and skills. This may be compounded by the fact that the same child also has difficulty concentrating on the related homework assignment. Consequently, the child may not be able to express whatever he or she has learned. Indecision would become a liability whenever a child had to choose between answers or between various courses of action that could be followed to complete schoolwork. This indecision would slow the child down when he or she is taking tests or completing assignments. The child who experiences fatigue isn't going to have the energy necessary to put forth a concerted effort in school or on homework. This child might tire out before completing assignments and thus fail to turn them in. Psychomotor retardation could affect a child academically by slowing his or her reaction times and movements such as writing, turning pages, or getting needed materials. In contrast, the child who is experiencing psychomotor agitation is moving so quickly and frequently that he or she can't sit still long enough to concentrate or complete work.

Evidence indicates that depressed children exhibit problems in school performance (Hollon, 1970; Stark, Livingston, et al., 1990). Brumback et al. (1977) investigated the relationship between depression and school performance among children who were referred to an Educational Diagnostic Center. Fifty-eight percent of the children were depressed. Of the depressed children, 71% evidenced a change in school performance, and 62% reported a change in attitude toward school that coincided with the occurrence of the depressive episode. In addition, 41% experienced school refusal during the depressive episode. Weinberg et al. (1973) also reported that 71% of their population of depressed children evidenced a change in school performance. They also reported that school refusal occurred more frequently during depressive episodes. Carlson and Cantwell (1979) reported that 48% of their depressed sample exhibited a decrease in school performance. This percentage was greater than that found among children with other psychological disorders.

Investigators have tried to determine whether depression is associated with a reduction in achievement in basic academic skills such as reading, spelling, and arithmetic as well as actual academic performance in the classroom. Results of the research are quite inconsistent. Tesiny, Lefkowitz, and Gordon (1980) reported a modest correlation between depression as assessed with a peer nomination inventory and reading ($r = -.23$) and math ($r = -.27$) achievement. Using a similar methodology, Lefkowitz and Tesiny (1985) reported a significant although modest correlation between depression and reading ($r = -.27$) and math ($r = -.33$) achievement among girls, but there was no relationship for boys. Vincenzi (1987) reported a significant relationship between depression as assessed with the CDI and a standardized measure of reading achievement ($r = -.40$). In contrast to these significant results, Strauss, Lahey, and Jacobsen (1982) did not find any significant relationship between depression as assessed with either the CDI or a peer nomination inventory of depression and achievement in reading or math when IQ was controlled. Similarly, Brumback, Jackoway, and Weinberg (1980) found no difference between depressed and nondepressed children in their achievement on a standardized measure of reading, spelling, or arithmetic. The authors concluded that the poor school performance of depressed children was not a cause of their depression, nor did it produce a reduction in their basic academic skills. Rather, the poor school performance was the result of depression-related disinterest in participation and self-deprecatory ideation.

The author's own research (see Stark, Livingston, et al., 1990) tends to be consistent with the two aforementioned studies. Results indicated that there were no significant differences between depressed and nondepressed controls on 13 of the 15 tests that comprise the California Achievement Test. The depressed children scored significantly lower than the controls on the Math Total and Social Studies test. When the scores of depressed children were compared to those of anxious children, the depressed children scored significantly lower on the Reading Vocabulary, Math Concepts and Applications, and on the Math Total tests. These differences in part resulted from the fact that the anxious children tended to receive the highest scores of the three diagnostic groups.

In a couple of investigations, researchers have attempted to determine the relationship between depression and actual achievement in school as reflected in GPA. Vincenzi (1987) reported a modest correlation between severity of depression and GPA ($r = -.26$). In the author's research (Stark, Livingston, et al., 1990), depressed children relative to controls had a significantly lower overall GPA and significantly lower grades in science, physical education, and language. In addition, depressed children had a significantly lower overall GPA and science grade than did anxious children. Puig-Antich et al. (1985a) completed an investigation of the effects of depression on academic achievement that included endogenous and nonendogenous depressed children, a psychiatric control group of other neurotic disordered children, and a normal control group. According to the children's mothers, children across all three psychiatric conditions were achieving in school at a significantly lower rate of performance relative to the normal controls. The endogenously depressed children were most severely impaired, followed by the psychiatric controls and then the nonendogenously depressed children. However, these differences were not statistically significant. When specific areas of achievement were analyzed, including reading, spelling, and arithmetic, a similar pattern of results emerged. The authors concluded that a disturbance in academic achievement existed but was nonspecific to psychological disturbance.

In a follow-up study, Puig-Antich et al. (1985b) evaluated the change in academic achievement that followed recovery from a depressive episode. Four months after successful treatment with antidepressant medication, the children's mothers reported a significant improvement in school achievement. In fact, according to their mothers they had improved to the point that they were rated similarly to the normal controls and significantly better than the nondepressed neurotic children. When these results are considered in combination with the earlier results of Puig-Antich et al. (1985a), it is apparent that, from a mother's perspective, psychological disorders are associated with a reduction in school achievement, and in the case of depression, the academic performance quickly returns to a normal level following successful treatment with antidepressant medication. It is important to note that the results of the Puig-Antich et al. studies are limited by the fact that the measure of academic achievement was based on the mothers' perceptions of their children's school performance. These perceptions may or may not be accurate for a variety of reasons.

To better understand the impairment in academic achievement associated with depression in children, a number of investigators have studied the relationship between depression and general and specific intellectual abilities. The investigators who have administered an entire intelligence test have not found any significant differences in the general intellectual ability of depressed and nondepressed youths. Leon, Kendall, and Garber (1980) assessed intelligence with the Peabody Picture Vocabulary Test and depression with the Personality Inventory for Children (Wirt et al., 1977). The authors did not report a significant difference in the IQs of the depressed and nondepressed youths. Kashani et al. (1983) administered the Wechsler Intelligence Scale for Children — Revised (WISC-R) to a sample of depressed and nondepressed children. They reported no significant difference between the two groups in either the full-scale, verbal, or performance IQs of the depressed and nondepressed children. Thus, it does not appear as though depression has a discernible adverse impact on general intellectual ability (as assessed with the PPVT and WISC-R), nor does subaverage intelligence appear to be the cause of depression in children.

Researchers have also explored the relationship between specific intellectual abilities, as assessed with various subtests of the WISC-R, and depression in children. Results have been inconsistent. Kaslow, Rehm, and Siegel (1984) hypothesized that depression would selectively impact some of the more complex nonverbal abilities assessed by certain subtests of the WISC-R while it would not affect verbal ability. More specifically, the authors predicted a relationship between depression and the Block Design, Digit Span, and Coding subtests, and they hypothesized that there would not be a significant relationship between depression and the Vocabulary subtest of the WISC-R. As the authors predicted, there was a significant negative correlation between scores on the CDI and the Block Design ($r = -.24$), Digit Span ($r = -.31$), and Coding ($r = -.22$) subtests. In contrast to the results on the nonverbal subtests, Kaslow and colleagues did not find a significant relationship between scores on the CDI and the Vocabulary subtest. Kaslow et al. (1983) partially replicated these results and extended them by including an anagrams test. Overall, on the anagrams test the children with higher CDI scores tended to complete fewer problems because they worked at a slower pace.

In contrast to the results of Kaslow and colleagues, McGee, Anderson, Williams, and Silva (1986) failed to find a significant relationship between depression and any of the subscales of the WISC-R. Thus, these investigators failed to find the relationship between depression and intellectual performance on the Block Design, Coding, and Digit Span subtests. Nor did they find that the performances of children on other subscales were adversely affected by depression.

The discrepancy in the results of these two groups of investigators may stem from their differing assessment methodologies. Kaslow and colleagues relied on the CDI as the sole measure of depression, whereas McGee and co-workers utilized a semi-structured interview to assess depression. This latter procedure is a much better assessment methodology, as it enables the investigator to select a sample of subjects who truly are depressed, whereas children who endorse depressive symptomatology on the CDI may have a variety of learning or psychological disturbances or no disorder at all (Stark, Kendall, & Rouse, 1990). This problem with false positives is exacerbated when a lower (less symptomatic) cut-off score is utilized to classify children as depressed on the CDI. The score utilized by Kaslow et al. (1983, 1984) led to approximately 30% of the sample of school children being classified as exhibiting significant levels of depressive symptomatology. As evident from the previous section of this chapter, this clearly is not the case.

A couple of investigators have studied the impact of one aspect of depression, negative affect, on learning among children. In general, the results of these studies indicate that induced negative affect has an adverse impact on the learning of preschool children in academic-like tasks. Masters, Barden, and Ford (1979) reported that negative affect decreased learning rates and slowed the performance of 4-year-old children on a shape discrimination learning task. Positive affect, in contrast, enhanced learning and rate of performance. On a letter discrimination task, induced negative affect increased the response latency and errors of 4- to 6-year-old children (Graves & Lahey, 1982). These results suggest that negative affect may impair some of the basic learning processes of children. However, more research is needed, and if this has application to depression, then it should be apparent when depressed and nondepressed children are compared to one another on similar tasks.

FAMILY INTERACTIONS AND
CHILDHOOD DEPRESSION

Numerous theories of childhood psychopathology emphasize the role of the family in the development and maintenance of psychological disorders. Given the central role of the family in these theories, it would seem logical that there would be a good deal of relevant research. Unfortunately, this is not the case. There is in fact a minimum of family-related research. In this section of the chapter, the literature related to the nature of the interactions of families with a depressed child will be reviewed. Included in this review will be a discussion of the impressions and observations of clinicians that have been published as well as relevant research that has been completed with depressed youths and their families.

Clinical Impressions

A number of clinician–researchers have described their impressions and observations of the interactions and relationships of families with a depressed child. In these articles, it is difficult to distinguish between the theoretical assumptions of the author and his or her observations, which is not surprising since the areas naturally color each other. A clinician is likely to conceptualize cases from a preferred theoretical perspective that leads him or her to look for, see, and label psychological phenomena in a specific way. Likewise, through actual clinical experience, an individual's theoretical scheme may be reinforced or altered. Given the complex nature of interpersonal interactions, the multitude of subtle and not so subtle behaviors, communications, and emotional reactions, it seems as though it would be possible for a clinician–researcher to find just about whatever he or she was looking for. Thus, it is important to read the following brief review with these aforementioned thoughts in mind as well as with an eye toward integration with the reader's own perspective.

Arieti and Bemporad (1980) paint a disturbing picture of the interactions of families with a depressed child. From their experiences, the power in the family typically lies with one dominant parent who is highly critical and intolerant of behavior that deviates from parental norms. The dominant parent uses punitive and psychologically damaging means such as guilt, shame, and threats of abandonment to enforce his or her rules and to coerce other family members into a submissive posture. Affection for a child is expressed contingently upon parental expectations for achievement and good behavior. The severity of the depressive disorder appeared to be related to which parent was dominant in the family. More severe depression was associated with maternal dominance, whereas paternal dominance was associated with moderate levels of depression.

Grossman, Poznanski, and Banegas (1983) have described their observations of parent–child interactions during lunchtime in a psychiatric clinic. Five of the families had a child who had received a diagnosis of a mood disorder. There were a couple of observations of these families that are relevant to this chapter. First, in two of the families with a depressed child, the mothers were "oversolicitous" of their daughters, focusing the entire conversation on them. Second, the authors noted that in the case where both parents were present with the depressed child, the disturbance in the marital relationship was expressed openly in front of the child, who appeared to be trying to split the parents apart.

Poznanski and Zrull (1970) reviewed the case notes of 14 depressed children aged 3 to 12 years. The authors identified a number of commonalities in the descriptions of their families. There was a relatively high rate of depression among the parents of the depressed children. The parents had difficulty handling aggression and hostility, and directed these emotions toward the helpless child. They frequently had temper outbursts and employed severe, punitive disciplinary techniques. When the child misbehaved, he or she was rejected. The parents also failed to support the child when he or she had difficulties mastering a situation. Thus, once again the child felt rejected. There were signs of rejection of the child, including abuse, neglect of the child's emotional and survival needs, and overt statements of rejection.

Kashani, Venzke, et al. (1981) interviewed 23 depressed children who were hospitalized for medical problems and their parents. During the interviews, systematic information was collected about the parents and the nature of the relationships among family members. In 20 cases, the parents reported their own emotional problems and difficulty adjusting to their child's "handicapping" condition. In addition, there was a greater frequency of intense marital discord reported compared to the rate found among the parents of nondepressed medical patients.

The authors identified a number of maladaptive patterns of behavior that occurred more frequently among families with a depressed child. More specifically the parents were excessively critical of the children, frequently finding faults with their youngster. The parents also teased their child and in some cases were extremely overprotective. When these three patterns of behavior are considered in combination, they would send the child the message that he or she was an unacceptable and inadequate person who could not function without parental supervision. This message, if internalized, would lead to a negative sense of self.

In the most objectively written case studies, Kashani and colleagues (Kashani & Carlson, 1987; Kashani, Ray, & Carlson, 1984) described the environments and relationships of families with a depressed preschool-age child. Depression is extremely rare among children this age (Kashani & Ray, 1985) and appears to be associated with family environments that are characterized by extreme chaos, neglect, family violence, parental psychopathology, and substance abuse by one or both parents. One of the depressed children clearly experienced the neglect of her basic needs, and the other four may have experienced emotional neglect as a result of parental psychopathology. In fact, all five of the mothers were experiencing some type of a psychological disorder. Four of the mothers were depressed, and one received a diagnosis of antisocial personality. One of the mothers had attempted suicide four times, and one of the fathers had committed suicide. Three of the children's natural fathers were alcoholics, and one mother abused drugs. The depressed child had been physically abused in three of the families, and there was evidence of "family violence" in another case. In addition to being physically abused, one of the depressed children had been sexually abused. Two of the mothers also had been abused by their husbands. Little information was given about the interaction patterns between the children and their mothers. However, in one case it was noted that the child was rejected by her mother, who ignored her behavior, including potentially dangerous behaviors. The child reciprocated by ignoring the mother's commands and attempts to initiate a conversation.

Pfeffer (1981) described her observations and theoretical opinions about families with suicidal children. Although it is recognized that not all suicidal children are depressed and not all depressed children are suicidal, there is a fair amount of overlap in these two populations. Thus, there may be something to be learned about families with a depressed youth from Pfeffer's years of experience with the families of suicidal children. Pfeffer noted that the family system with a suicidal child was characterized by vaguely defined generational boundaries, serious marital conflicts, symbiotic parent–child relationships, projection of parental feelings onto the child, and inflexibility in this pattern. The parents were self-indulgent in a regressive way that excluded the child's needs or desires. Change in the pattern was viewed as a threat to the survival of the family. On a more emotional level, the family interactions were often vague and hostile, with little expression of empathy or support. Overall, this pattern of interactions, which was intense, fixed, and of long duration, prevented the children's progress toward individuation and autonomy.

Empirical Investigations

There are very few existing empirical studies of the relationships and interactions of families with a depressed youngster. Results of the existing investigations do not create a clear picture of the parent–

child interactions and relationships associated with childhood depression. However, as will become apparent, there are some consistencies across studies, and, in general, the evidence indicates that there are maladaptive interaction patterns among families with a psychologically disturbed youngster.

Amanat and Butler (1984) compared the interactions of the families with a depressed child to those with an overanxious child. Their methodology was noteworthy since they have completed one of the few studies in which the family was actually observed while interacting. The entire family completed a decision-making task. In addition, each parent completed an "oppressive behavior" questionnaire. Results of the observations revealed that there were no significant differences between the groups in the parental coalition, hierarchy of power, or self-expression of the parents. There were significant differences between the groups in the amount of control exerted by the parents over the children. The parents of depressed children, unlike the parents of the overanxious children, tended to be dominant and exerted nearly total control over the decision-making process. In the majority of cases, the children's attempts at self-expression and autonomy were suppressed by the parents of the depressed children during the decision-making task, thus forcing them into a submissive, helpless posture.

Results of the oppressive behavior questionnaire were consistent in many ways with the parents' behavior during the decision-making task. The parents who had a depressed child indicated a greater tendency to control their child's decisions and behavior through oppressive means. Furthermore, the parents indicated a preference for friends who would not threaten the parents' authority. No differences were found between the parents of the two groups in terms of invasiveness, intrusion into the children's self-expressions, empathy with the children's needs, or attitudes toward chores or time/space needs. However, since this study did not include a normal control group, it was not possible to determine whether the families with a depressed child deviated from families with psychologically healthy children. It also is important to note that since the two pathological groups did not differ from each other on some of the characteristics, if a normal control group had been included, and if the two pathological groups differed from them, this still would indicate that these were characteristics that were nonspecific to the type of psychological disorder.

Kaslow and colleagues (1984) conducted a study of the self-control skills of mildly depressed school children. The primary results supported the viability of Rehm's (1977) self-control model of depression. The authors also made a preliminary attempt to determine whether there was a difference between children who endorsed elevated levels of depressive symptomatology and nondepressed children in their perceptions of their families. The children were asked to complete an eight-item questionnaire that the authors developed specifically for this investigation. The children who endorsed elevated levels of depressive symptomatology, relative to normal controls, reported significantly more dysfunction in their families. However, the exact nature of the dysfunction was not reported, nor would that have been possible with the measure that was utilized.

As part of a study of the correlates of childhood depression, Lefkowitz and Tesiny (1985) explored the relationship between maternal rejection and marital disharmony, and depression among their children. Depression was assessed through a peer nomination inventory, and the family-related variables were assessed through an interview of the 508 mothers who participated. Results indicated a modest relationship ($r = .33$) between maternal rejection and childhood depression. Curiously, results for the analyses on the marital disharmony section of the interview were not reported.

Asarnow and associates (Asarnow, Carlson, & Guthrie, 1987) compared the perceptions of the family environments of children who were diagnosed as depressed, suicidal, or suffering from other nonpsychotic psychological disorders. The latter group of subjects ($n = 13$) served as a psychiatric control group. The authors did not include a normal control group. Furthermore, there commonly was secondary coexisting pathology that overlapped with the primary disorders exhibited by the psychiatric control group. It also is important to note that it is not clear how many of the suicidal children also were depressed or experiencing some other psychological disorder. The 30 youngsters, who were inpatients in a neuropsychiatric institute, completed a number of self-report measures including a portion of the Family Environment Scale (FES; Moos & Moos, 1981). The children completed five subscales including three that comprised the interpersonal relationship domain (Cohesion, Expressiveness, Conflict) and two that comprised the system maintenance domain (Organization, Control).

Results of the study indicated that there were no differences between the perceptions of the depressed children and the psychiatric control subjects on these five subscales and the two broader domains. In contrast, the suicidal children perceived their families as being significantly less cohesive, higher in conflict, and less controlled. Once again it was not possible to determine whether depressed children perceived their family milieu to be different from that of normal children. Furthermore, given the small sample size and the fact that the depressed group was not homogeneous, it is not surprising that there were no significant differences between subjects from these two groups. A more sensitive measure may be required to find the more subtle differences that might exist between these two groups. Suicide is considered to be a statement that the youngster is experiencing an intolerable situation from which he or she can see no other escape. Thus, it would seem logical that these youngsters would report a significantly more disturbed family environment. Nevertheless, the results do indicate that there are some characteristics of the family environment that may be related to suicide among children.

Stark and colleagues (Stark, Humphrey, Crook, & Lewis, 1990) compared children's and mothers' perceptions of the environments of families with a depressed, anxious, or normal control child. Participants in the study were 51 school children from grades four through seven and their maternal figures ($n = 43$). The children were diagnosed as having a depressive, anxiety, or mixed disorder with the K-SADS (Puig-Antich & Ryan, 1986), and they completed the children's version of the Self-Report Measure of Family Functioning (SRMFF-C; Stark, Humphrey, et al., 1990). Results of this study clearly indicated that there were significant disturbances in the perceived family environments of children with a depressive or anxiety disorder. The greatest disturbance was found among families with a depressed child. Families with a depressed or anxious child are characterized by the affected child as less cohesive, more conflictual, and less open to expression of any type. In addition, the parents of these children manage their families through more autocratic means, allowing the children minimal input into decision making. All of these factors seem to combine and contribute to a sense of dissatisfaction with the family.

Families of children with depressive disorders also were characterized by lower levels of activity of a social, recreational, or intellectual/cultural nature. Since the families are more restricted in their involvement in such pleasant activities, the children have fewer opportunities to receive positive reinforcement from involvement in them. In addition, they have fewer opportunities to escape from what they perceive to be a conflictual and stifling environment. Failure to get involved in pleasant activities leaves the depressed child to sit around and get lost in his or her depressive thinking, which simply exacerbates the problem. In addition, it contributes to the lethargy and lack of inertia expressed by depressed youths. Since many depressed children come from abusive and chaotic environments, this failure to get involved in activities eliminates a potential buffer to the impact of this environment: contact with a healthier and supportive external world. This may be equally true of families with a psychologically impaired parent. By the restriction of external contact, the child is trapped with the parent. Finally, failure to engage in recreational, social, and cultural activities leads to a diminished opportunity to develop psychosocially and to develop a sense of personal efficacy as one masters his or her world.

The greatest level of overt conflict in the family was reported by depressed children. It appears as though there is a growing body of research (see Forehand et al., 1988; Puig-Antich et al., 1985a) that implicates family conflict as being a psychologically destructive force. From existing research it is not possible to determine the source of the family conflict. It is not clear whether the conflict is between the parents, the parents and the child, the child and a sibling, a sibling and the parents, or some other combination of combatants. Nevertheless, conflict in the family, regardless of its source and direction, could leave a child feeling angry, insecure, guilty, and possibly afraid to express him- or herself because of fear of provoking a conflict. If the conflict is directed toward the child, he or she could perceive a message of rejection and devaluation that could lead to a negative sense of the self. If the household as a whole is characterized by conflict, the child could develop a sense of the world as being a hostile place. Furthermore, it could lead to a sense of hopelessness as the child fails to initiate change-producing actions because "they'll just get mad at me, so why bother to try?"

Results of discriminant function analyses computed on the children's responses to the SRMFF-C indicated that 68% of the children could be accurately classified into their diagnostic groups.

Results of the ratings on the SRMFF completed by mothers were less robust. With the exception of family involvement in recreational activities, mothers of depressed children and anxious children rated their families as similar to those with control children. Once again, families with a depressed child tended to be less involved in recreational activities, which confirms the child's perceptions. Although there were few significant differences among the groups based on mothers' ratings, according to the results of discriminant function analyses, their ratings on the SRMFF accurately predicted the diagnostic group membership of 71% of the depressed children and 78% of the anxious children.

Cole and Rehm (1986) explored parental variables that might contribute to the development of the deficits in self-control skills exhibited by depressed children. Subjects in the study were depressed ($n = 15$) and nondepressed inpatients ($n = 15$) and nonclinic nondepressed ($n = 15$) children 8- to 12-years-old and their mothers and fathers. Each participant completed a standards-setting questionnaire and a measure of rewards and punishments. In addition, the triad participated in a family interaction task in which the child played a challenging game, and the parents were instructed to help the child in any way they wanted except for completing the task themselves. A circumscribed set of codes was used to quantify the interactions of the triad including: (1) child's performance on the game; (2) maternal rewards and maternal punishment; (3) paternal rewards and paternal punishment; and (4) self-reward and self-punishment.

Partial support was obtained for the hypothesis that the self-control deficits exhibited by depressed children were a reflection of the possible internalization of the excessively stringent expectations of their mothers. The parents, and mothers in particular, of depressed children set high standards for their children's performance and only expressed positive affect (social rewards) when their children's performance reached these higher levels of achievement. It is important to note that there was no difference in parental standards across diagnostic groups. In fact, it appeared as though parents, regardless of their child's diagnostic disposition, set high standards for their child's performance. However, the pattern of high expectations and minimal expression of positive affect was in part an expression of the mother's depression. In contrast, the mothers of nonclinic nondepressed children tended to express positive affect (social rewards) over a broader range of performance including the lower and moderate levels. Thus, it appeared as though the depressed children had to perform for longer periods of time without receiving any positive messages from their parents, and they would only receive positive expressions of affect on attainment of very high levels of performance.

Depressed children also set high standards for their own performance and only reduced the number of negative expressions on attainment of these elevated levels of performance. It also is important to note that there was no difference between depressed and normal groups in terms of the standards of performance set by the children. Rather, the differences were in the amounts of reinforcement they self-administered at lower and moderate levels of performance.

In the most comprehensive studies of the relationships among families with a depressed child, Puig-Antich and colleagues (1985a, 1985b) explored the nature of the mother–child, father–child, and marital relationships during an episode of major depression and 4 months following recovery from the episode. The results of their first investigation (Puig-Antich et al., 1985a) indicated that from the perspectives of the mothers with a depressed child, relative to normal controls, there were disruptions in all of the social relationships addressed in this investigation. Some of these disturbances appeared to be specific to the depressive disorder, whereas others appeared to be nonspecific to psychological disorders.

The mother in the mother–child relationship that contains children with major depression and other neurotic psychological disorders was characterized as impaired. And the greatest impairment resulting from this could be found among endogenously depressed youngsters, followed by neurotically depressed children, and then a control group of children with other neurotic disorders. The mothers of children with psychological disorders relative to those with normal children reported less communication with their psychologically disturbed child, and the communication they did have was described as being of poorer quality. The mothers' relationships with their impaired child were cold, hostile, tense, and sometimes rejecting. Mother–child dyads with a depressed youngster did not engage in as many activities together as did mother–child dyads with normal children. In addition, depressed children and children who had other neurotic disorders experienced more severe punishment. The pattern of results indicated that the impairments in communication and in the affective tone of the relationship were specific to depression, since mothers of children in both depressed groups reported significantly more impairment than did mothers of children with other neurotic disorders and normal children.

Mothers also completed interview ratings of the father–child relationship. In general, the results were similar to those of the mother–child relationship except that the differences among groups were of a lesser magnitude, which resulted in fewer significant between-groups differences. Significantly less communication was reported for psychologically impaired children relative to normal controls, and the quality of the communication was rated lower. The father–child relationship was cooler, more hostile, and tense in families with a psychologically disturbed child relative to families with normal children. There were no significant differences between the depressed and neurotic disorders control group. Thus, in the case of the father–child relationship, the differences appeared to be nonspecific to psychological disorder. There were no significant differences between any of the groups in number of activities engaged in or limits set.

The marital relationship was explored in detail from the mother's perspective. There were no significant differences between groups in irritability, complaining, quarrels, activities together, whole-family activities together, affection, satisfaction, conversations together, problem-solving and decision-making styles, sharing of housework, global warmth, or hostility. The sole significant between-group difference was in disagreements about child rearing, which appeared to be specific to the depressive disorders groups.

Puig-Antich and colleagues (1985a) concluded that the disturbances in interpersonal relations were most likely a result of the disorder itself rather than the psychosocial milieu. The affective symptoms of dysphoric and angry mood could produce the cold and hostile tenor of the parent–child relationships. The disruptions in quantity and quality of communication could be caused by the symptoms of social withdrawal, lack of concentration, and fatigue as well as psychomotor retardation.

In a second study, Puig-Antich and colleagues (1985b) used the same interview with mothers that they used in the aforementioned study to determine whether there were any changes in social relations following reductions in depressive symptoms. The interview was completed with the mothers 4 months after their children's depressive episode had remitted. In general, the amount of improvement in a specific aspect of psychosocial relations was related to the severity of the disruption in that aspect of the relationship during the depressive episode. More specifically, the more severe the disruption, the smaller the improvement following termination of the depressive episode. The aspects of psychosocial functioning that were most impaired during the episode either took longer to recover or only partially recovered.

The most noticeable changes were in the mother–child relationship, where mothers reported a significant improvement in the quantity and quality of communication. The negative affect associated with their interactions with the depressed youngster also decreased. In addition, the severity of the punishment administered by the mothers was significantly reduced. Mothers only reported one statistically significant improvement in the father–child relationship: the quantity of communications significantly increased. There were no significant changes in the marital relationship.

The authors concluded that a depressive episode in a child may act as a superimposed agent producing or exacerbating deficits and distortions in the family relationships especially the mother–child relationship. These deficits and distortions probably are reversible. The affective state of the depressed child may be the central contributor to many of the psychological difficulties in which he or she is involved.

TREATMENT OUTCOME RESEARCH

Overview

The review of treatment outcome research that follows includes brief summaries of all of the existing published investigations of which the author is aware. Readers may find the dearth of studies surprising and maybe unbelievable given the severity and prevalence of depression among children. The reasons are unclear for the paucity of systematic research. However, it may stem from the fact that the very existence of a depressive disorder among children was denied in the recent past, and more recently its existence and nature was a subject of debate. It was not until 1980 that depression was recognized as a clinical disorder among children by the American Psychiatric Association. Another possible reason is the fact that a psychometrically sound assessment methodology just began to appear in the last 6 years (Reynolds, 1984).

The review will cover a pair of behaviorally oriented case studies and two control group treatment investigations that were conducted in the schools with moderately depressed youths. There are a few psychoanalytically oriented case reports in the literature (Furman, 1974; Sacks, 1977), but they will not be discussed because of the failure to employ an empirical methodology and because the procedures that were employed were not stated in a manner possible to replicate. The author's research that serves as the empirical base for the treatment program described in a later section of this book will be discussed in some detail.

Behaviorally Oriented Investigations

Petti and colleagues (Petti, Bornstein, Delamater, & Conner, 1980) described a multimodal treatment for a 10½ year-old girl who was hospitalized for chronic, severe dysphoria. She was referred for depression, educational difficulties, and an evaluation of her suitability for foster placement. The patient's natural parents were chronic alcoholics who may have abused her. She was experiencing difficulties in her foster placement, was exhibiting minor antisocial behavior, and did not have any social relationships. During the course of treatment, the patient was evaluated by the hospital staff twice a day using the Children's Behavior Inventory (CBI; Burdock & Hardesty, 1964) and the Scale of School Age Depression (SSAD) to determine the effectiveness of the treatment program. The treatment program consisted of four primary modes of therapy including individual, group, family, and pharmacological. The initial regimen of individual psychotherapy consisted of using the therapeutic relationship to help her understand her feelings about her natural and foster parents and to improve her self-image. In addition, an individualized teaching program was developed and utilized to remediate her educational deficiencies and thus improve her self-esteem. The group treatment consisted of a creative dramatics group that was used as an outlet for her feelings, a means of giving and receiving feedback, and as an arena for testing new behaviors. Concurrent to the individual and group treatment, the patient and her foster family were involved in family therapy that was designed to facilitate the development of a more adaptive environment for her eventual return. A number of additional sessions were held between the child and her natural mother.

This comprehensive treatment regimen did not produce any noticeable improvement in her hospital behavior as assessed with the CBI and SSAD. Consequently, imipramine (an antidepressant medication) treatment was initiated, which produced a marked improvement in her overt signs of anger, a decrease in fears and worries, and an improvement in depressive behaviors. She also reported feeling happier. The authors believed that the imipramine also made her more amenable to the psychological interventions that followed.

The final treatment component was social-skills training. This training consisted of education, modeling, rehearsal, and feedback that was used to teach the patient to increase the amount of eye contact, the frequency and duration of smiles, duration of speech, and number of requests for new behaviors from others. Treatment was conducted in nine 15-minute sessions over 3 weeks. The skills training was successful at producing a "marked" improvement in the target behaviors. The child was eventually discharged from the hospital, and both the child and her foster mother reported a maintenance of improvements at a 6-week check-up.

In another behaviorally oriented case study, Frame, Matson, Sonis, Fialkov, and Kazdin (1982) described the treatment of a 10-year-old boy who had been hospitalized for major depression, suicidal ideation and gestures, poor school performance, and violent temper outbursts. The diagnosis of major depression was based on both the mother's report and an independent rater's evaluation. The treatment was complicated by the fact that the child had an IQ of 79.

A number of overt behaviors were identified by the authors for modification, including poor eye contact, inaudible speech, one-word answers, bland facial expressions, and body position indicative of social withdrawal. The treatment consisted of instruction, modeling, rehearsal, and feedback. The training was conducted daily (every weekday) for 20 minutes at a time. The targets of the first six sessions were body position and eye contact, which were worked on simultaneously. Speech quality was the focus of the next five sessions. The final nine sessions were spent working on the expression of affect.

A multiple-baseline design across the three phases of treatment was used to evaluate the efficacy of the behavioral training. Each behavior systematically improved when treatment was introduced. Twelve weeks after treatment, the improvements were still evident. Although these changes appear to provide support for the efficacy of this approach to the treatment of depression, the authors provided a caveat. They noted that the behaviors that were targeted for change were nonspecific to depression. The target behaviors are evident in children with a variety of behavioral disorders. Since they did not assess for the syndrome of depression at pretreatment and posttreatment, there was no evidence that the syndrome of depression (emotional, cognitive, motivational, and vegetative symptoms) had changed.

In response to the concerns of school personnel, Butler, Miezitis, Friedman, and Cole (1980) developed and empirically evaluated two treatment programs for depressed youths. The participants in this investigation were 56 children from public schools including 35 boys and 21 girls from grades 5 and 6. The children were identified through a two-step procedure that consisted of first identifying the children through an assessment battery and then checking with the children's teachers to verify that they were exhibiting depressive behavior in the classroom. The assessments were conducted at pretreatment and again at posttreatment. The assessment battery consisted of the CDI (Kovacs, 1981), Piers–Harris Children's Self-Concept Scale (Piers, 1969), Moyal–Miezitis Stimulus Appraisal Questionnaire (Moyal, 1977), the Nowicki–Strickland Locus of Control Scale for Children (Nowicki & Strickland, 1973), and an unstructured interview of each child's teacher.

The children were assigned randomly to one of four experimental conditions including a role-play treatment, a cognitive restructuring treatment, attention placebo control, and waiting list control condition. Children in the two active treatments and the attention placebo condition met 10 times, once a week, in groups of six to eight children for an hour each time.

The role-play (RP) treatment consisted of training in a number of behavioral and cognitive skills. At the behavioral level, the children were taught social skills. At the cognitive level, the children were sensitized to their thoughts and feelings as well as those of others. In addition, the children were taught the problem-solving skill of generating alternatives when facing stressful or threatening situations. The skills were taught through role plays followed by discussion and then additional role plays. In addition, the children were given therapeutic homework assignments.

The cognitive restructuring (CR) treatment was designed to teach the children the relationship between thoughts and feelings and to identify maladaptive thoughts and then to adopt more adaptive ones. In addition, the children were taught listening skills, and they were given therapeutic homework assignments. The training procedure used with children in this group consisted of the didactic presentation of the treatment material. The authors noted that this treatment program did not have the "appeal" of the RP program. Since treatment involvement is one of the best predictors of treatment outcome with children (Braswell, Kendall, Braith, Carey, & Uye, 1985), this is a major problem for this particular intervention.

Children in the attention placebo (AP) condition were taught to solve academic problems as a group through sharing research and pooling information. Children in the waiting list (WL) condition simply completed the assessment battery at pre- and posttreatment assessments.

Results of the investigation indicated that children in all four experimental conditions reported significant improvement on the CDI at the posttreatment assessment. Children who received the RP treatment also reported significant improvements from pretreatment to posttreatment on the measures of self-esteem, locus of control, and stimulus appraisal. In contrast to these very favorable results, children who received the CR treatment reported a significant improvement in self-esteem, and the children in the two control groups did *not* report any significant improvement in self-esteem, locus of control, or stimulus appraisal. Following treatment, each child's teacher was interviewed to determine whether he or she noticed any change in the child's depressive behaviors. The teacher's perceptions were quite consistent with those of the children. Teachers reported improvement in 9 of 14 children in the RP condition, 4 of 14 in the CR condition, 3 of 14 in the AP condition, and 2 of 14 in the WL condition. The authors noted a potential confounding variable that may have contributed to the improvement noted in the three children in the AP and two children in the WL conditions. These children had participated in a special three-session resource program that was designed to improve social relationships.

Reynolds and Coats (1986) evaluated the relative efficacy of cognitive–behavioral therapy (CBT) and relaxation training (RT) for the treatment of moderately depressed adolescents. Thirty youngsters with an average age of 15½ years were identified in their high schools through a multiple-gate assessment procedure (this assessment procedure is described in Chapter 3). Depression was measured at pretreatment, posttreatment, and 5-week follow-up assessments using multiple procedures including two self-report scales and a clinical interview. More specifically, the adolescents completed the Beck Depression Inventory (BDI; Beck et al., 1961), the Reynolds Adolescent Depression Scale (RADS; Reynolds, 1987a), and they were interviewed with the Bellevue Index of Depression (BID; Petti, 1978). The youngsters were randomly assigned to either the CBT, RT, or a waiting list (WL) control condition. The treatments were delivered in ten 50-minute sessions over a 5-week period. The participants met at their schools in groups of five with one therapist.

The CBT consisted of a combination of treatment components that have been successfully employed with depressed adults by Lewinsohn (see Zeiss, Lewinsohn, & Munoz, 1979) and Rehm (see Fuchs & Rehm, 1977). More specifically, the youngsters were taught a number of self-control skills including self-monitoring, self-evaluation, and self-reinforcement. The skills were taught through didactic presentations and extratherapy homework assignments. In addition, the self-control skills were combined and utilized in a self-change program.

The RT consisted of training in progressive muscle relaxation and work toward self-administered relaxation during stressful times. Progressive relaxation was taught and practiced during the treatment sessions and practiced at home and in stressful situations. Participants in the WL condition completed the assessment battery at pretreatment, posttreatment, and follow-up assessments.

The results of the investigation indicated that the CBT and RT treatments were equally effective at reducing depression across all three measures of depression at posttreatment assessment. In addition, subjects in both active treatments reported significant improvement in anxiety and academic self-concept. Qualitative analyses indicated that 83% of the adolescents in the CBT condition and 75% of the RT condition scored in the normal range on the BDI. The results on the BDI and BID were maintained at the 5-week follow-up assessment.

A Program of Treatment Outcome Research

In the first of the authors' treatment studies with depressed youths (Stark, Reynolds, & Kaslow, 1987), two treatment programs that were downward extensions of interventions for depressed adults were compared to each other and to a waiting list control condition. One of the treatments was based on Rehm's self-control therapy (Rehm, Kaslow, & Rabin, 1987), and the other was a behavioral intervention that was loosely based on Lewinsohn's treatment program (cf. Lewinsohn, Sullivan, & Grosscup, 1980).

Children in grades 4 to 6 from a public school were screened for depression using the CDI (Kovacs, 1981). The children who reported elevated levels of symptomatology (total score greater than 16) completed a more thorough assessment, which included a second administration of the CDI and a single administration of the Child Depression Scale (CDS; Reynolds, 1987b), a clinical interview entitled the Children's Depression Rating Scale — Revised (CDRS-R; Poznanski et al., 1984), a measure of self-esteem (Coopersmith, 1967), and anxiety (Reynolds & Richmond, 1985). Depression was also assessed from each child's mother's perspective with the Child Behavior Checklist (CBCL; Achenbach & Edelbrock, 1979). This assessment battery was completed at pretreatment, posttreatment, and at a 8-week follow-up.

The pretreatment assessment process identified 29 children who exhibited mild to moderate levels of depressive symptomatology across the self-report and interview measures of depression. These children were randomly assigned to one of the three experimental conditions. The treatments were conducted in the children's school in small groups of four or five. Both intervention programs consisted of twelve 45 to 50 minute meetings completed over 5 weeks.

The self-control treatment was designed to teach the children more adaptive skills for self-monitoring, self-evaluation, attributing the causes of various outcomes, and self-consequating. The skills were taught through didactic presentations and in-therapy activities, and they were applied through extratherapy homework assignments. In the later sessions, the skills were combined as a means of working toward self-improvement. Self-monitoring was taught during the first four sessions and was applied to the children's daily lives through the use of pleasant events schedules. These schedules were completed daily for the duration of the treatment program. To increase the probability that the children would complete their self-monitoring assignments and other homework, the children contracted for tangible rewards that were distributed by the therapists on an intermittent schedule. During sessions five and six, the focus of the self-monitoring was on the long-term rather than short-term consequences of their behavior.

The later portion of session six and all of session seven were devoted to teaching the youngsters a more adaptive attributional style. This was accomplished through education and role playing. Children were taught a more adaptive means of evaluating their own performances and abilities through a combination of an educational exercise and cognitive restructuring during sessions eight and nine. In addition, at this time the children began setting goals and subgoals for self-improvement, and they combined their new skills (self-monitoring, a new attributional style, and self-evaluating) in an attempt to work toward goal attainment. Overt and covert forms of self-reinforcement were taught during the final three sessions, and they were applied by the children to goal and subgoal attainment as they worked toward self-improvement.

The behavioral problem-solving therapy consisted of education about feelings and interpersonal behavior and a combination of training in problem-solving skills, self-monitoring of pleasant events, activity scheduling, and social-skills training. Self-monitoring and group problem solving were used to increase pleasant activity level. The skills were taught through didactic presentations and in-therapy exercises, and they were applied through extratherapy homework assignments. Once again, to help insure therapeutic compliance, these children contracted for the same tangible rewards that were administered on the same intermittent schedule utilized with the children in the self-control condition.

Children in the waiting list condition did not receive treatment until after the posttreatment assessments had been completed. However, during this time, they were not excluded from any services that they would have received through the special education referral process in their school. Two of the students from the waiting list condition were referred to the school psychologist, who met with them individually once a week for therapy.

Results of the study indicated that children in both treatment conditions reported a significant reduction in depression at posttesting across depression measures and reported significantly less depressive symptomatology than children in the waiting list condition. Children in the waiting list condition reported a minimum of change. A look at the clinical significance of the changes revealed that 78% of the children in the self-control treatment program and 60% of the children in the behavioral problem-solving treatment scored in the nondepressed range on the CDI, and all of the children scored in the nondepressed range on the CDRS-R. On the measures of anxiety and self-esteem, children in both groups reported a significant reduction in anxiety, but only children in the self-control treatment reported a significant improvement in self-esteem on the Coopersmith.

The results of the mothers' ratings on the Child Behavior Checklist were less clear. The mothers' ratings of their children's depression were not correlated with the children's self-ratings of depression at pretreatment. This issue of lack of agreement will be discussed in Chapter 3. Nonetheless, the mothers of children in the behavioral problem-solving condition reported a significant improvement on the internalizing scale and on the depression and social withdrawal subscales. However, there were no significant between-group differences.

The improvements noted by the children in both active treatments at posttesting were maintained at 5-week follow-up. In fact, children in the self-control condition continued to improve and reported significantly less depression than the children in the behavioral problem-solving condition on the interview at follow-up. In addition, they reported a significantly more positive level of self-esteem. In contrast, the mothers of children in the behavioral problem-solving condition relative to the mothers of children in the self-control condition reported significantly less social withdrawal and internalizing symptomatology on the Child Behavior Checklist.

The results of this initial investigation were encouraging and led to a second study that was designed to determine whether a multicomponent cognitive–behavioral treatment contributed anything to the psychological change process beyond the nonspecifics of psychotherapy. To accomplish this goal, the relative efficacy of a cognitive–behavioral treatment was compared to a nonspecific psychotherapy control condition.

Approximately 700 children from grades 4 to 7 were screened for depression with the CDI. The youngsters who scored 16 or higher on the initial screening completed a second administration of the CDI approximately 2 weeks later. Those children who once again scored 16 or higher were interviewed with the K-SADS, and they completed a measure of depressive cognitions, self-esteem, and hopelessness. As a result of this assessment process, 26 youngsters were identified who reported elevated levels of depressive symptomatology, including 3 who received diagnoses of major depression, 10 who received diagnoses of dysthymic disorder, 2 who received diagnoses of depressive disorder not otherwise specified, and 2 who received a diagnosis of adjustment disorder with depressed mood. The other nine children reported elevated levels of symptomatology as assessed with the K-SADS and CDI, but it was either not severe enough or not of long enough duration to warrant a diagnosis. These children and their parents were invited to participate in the treatment program. Two youngsters (both seventh graders) declined.

The 24 remaining children were randomly assigned to either a cognitive–behavioral treatment or a traditional counseling condition that controlled for the nonspecifics of psychotherapy. The treatments were conducted in school and at home with the child and his or her parents. The school portion of both treatments was conducted in small groups of four with a pair of therapists. The therapists were doctoral students in school psychology. Both programs consisted of 24–26 sessions lasting 45–50 minutes conducted over a 3½-month period. The groups met two times a week for 8 weeks and once a week thereafter. In addition to the group sessions, there were family meetings conducted once a month. These meetings were held at home and included the depressed child, his or her parents, and one of the therapists who colead the child's group at school. Each family meeting lasted between 1 and 1½ hours and was scheduled at the family's convenience.

The cognitive–behavioral treatment consisted of training in self-control skills, social skills, and cognitive restructuring. More specifically, the self-control training consisted of teaching the children more adaptive self-consequation, self-monitoring, and self-evaluation. Assertiveness training focused on interactions with significant others including asking someone to do something fun, giving positive feedback, and telling someone to stop doing something that is annoying. Social-skills training emphasized initiating interactions, maintaining interactions, and handling conflict. Relaxation training and imagery were used to help prepare the children for using their skills. Cognitive restructuring was employed by the therapists throughout treatment. Emphasis was placed on the children acquiring and self-initiating the use of the cognitive restructuring procedures. In addition to the daily use, a number of sessions were entirely devoted to the acquisition of the cognitive restructuring techniques. A couple of sessions were devoted to teaching the children general problem-solving strategies. The family sessions were designed to teach the parents how to encourage their child to use his or her new skills and to engage in more pleasant family activities.

The traditional counseling control condition was designed to control for the nonspecifics of psychotherapy as they relate to this study, including such things as meeting with a group of peers who have similar problems, meeting with warm and empathic adults, being given a rationale for what causes depression and how to overcome it, talking about problems, gaining a support group, being given the expectation that they will get better, the demand characteristics of the situation that pull for the children to say that they are feeling better, and completion of therapeutic exercises. These groups were more consistent with traditional views of group therapy. The therapists attempted to facilitate group process work. Thus, the group interactions, discussions, and suggestions served as the therapeutic vehicle. Each session the therapists also involved the children in an exercise that would either help them learn more about emotions and how they are expressed or in a self-esteem-enhancing exercise. When the children presented with a specific problem, the therapists brought it to the group's attention where it was discussed. The therapists worked in an empathic and nondirective fashion. They were specifically instructed not to knowingly employ any cognitive or behavioral procedures. The primary objective of the family sessions was improving communication and increasing engagement in pleasant family activities.

Results of a repeated-measures (pre–post) multivariate (K-SADS, ATQ, CDI) analysis of variance revealed a significant main effect for treatment, time, and measure. In addition, significant treatment-by-measure and time-by-measure interactions were found. Subsequent between- and within-groups differences were analyzed with t-tests. Results of the within-groups analyses indicated that subjects in both treatment conditions reported significantly less depression at posttesting relative to pretesting on both the K-SADS and CDI. Likewise, the youngsters reported significantly fewer depressive cognitions. Comparisons of the posttreatment and 7-month follow-up data indicated that the improvements were maintained. Perhaps of greater interest were the between-group analyses. Although there had been no significant between-group differences prior to treatment on any of the three measures, at posttreatment assessment, subjects in the cognitive–behavioral treatment reported significantly less depression on the K-SADS interview and significantly fewer depressive cognitions on the ATQ. There was no significant difference on the CDI. At 7-month follow-up assessment, the differences were no longer significant. This was in part because of attrition. Only five of the children from the traditional counseling condition could be found, and only seven of the children from the cognitive–behavioral group were located. The children's scores on the measures had not changed; rather, the composition of the groups had changed with a few of the children who had reported the most improvement at posttesting in the cognitive–behavioral group not being included at follow-up, and a few of the youngsters from the traditional counseling group who had reported the least improvement not being located at follow-up for participation.

Overall, the results were quite encouraging, since the changes were not only statistically significant but also clinically significant.

The differences between the groups were somewhat surprising, since the treatment programs were conducted by inexperienced graduate students who were more proficient at conducting groups in a more traditional format. The results suggest that the additional skills training that the subjects in the cognitive–behavioral group received added something to the efficacy of the treatment program. Which component or components were the necessary and sufficient ones to do this is not known and couldn't be determined from the design of the study. This remains a question for future research.

CONCLUSIONS

Depression adversely affects a relatively large number of children. The prevalence rates appear to vary for a variety of reasons. Within the general school population, figures vary from approximately 4% to 13.9%. Since our figure of 4% (Stark, Laurent, et al., 1990) was based on 3 years of research involving over 1,400 children, whereas the higher figure of 13.9% reported by Pfeffer et al. (1984) was based on an one-time sample of 100 children, it seems as though the lower figure is more likely to be accurate. Research also suggests that higher prevalence rates are found among children with learning problems and children with serious medical concerns. Furthermore, a substantial number of children referred to psychiatric hospitals are experiencing a depressive disorder. Something this research to date seems to overlook is the fact that most children do not experience depressive disorders in isolation. Rather, depression commonly co-occurs with other disorders, most commonly anxiety disorders. Thus, depression may be one part of a bigger clinical picture of psychological disturbance.

It appears as though depression has an adverse effect on a child's performance in school. The reason for the deficit is unclear. However, it probably is because of the debilitating effect of a number of the symptoms rather than an intellectual impairment. Especially problematic are difficulty concentrating, fatigue, negative self-evaluations, hopelessness, anhedonia, and psychomotor disturbances. There is some evidence (Puig-Antich et al., 1985b) that suggests that the deficit in performance is not a permanent one. Rather, the youngster's achievement in school seems to recover relatively quickly following recovery from the episode.

A child's family plays a very influential role in his or her psychosocial development. Research is just beginning to appear that explores the possible contribution of the family to the development of depression in children. Prior to summarizing the results of this literature, a couple of points need to be emphasized. At the outset it is important to recognize that all of the research to date has been limited in a number of ways. First, there has been a paucity of observational studies. Future investigations should adopt this more costly, although richer methodology. Second, the research has tended to be unidirectional in nature. Thus, it has failed to evaluate the depressed child's role in the development and maintenance of the disturbances in family interactions. Third, there probably is no single pattern of disturbance in family interactions that leads to depression. Rather, a variety of possible avenues can be taken, all of which culminate in a child who is prone to experiencing depression. Finally, I would like to emphasize the fact that over the years we have worked with many depressed children who come from families that, while they are experiencing the natural distress surrounding the reality of having a disturbed child, are quite healthy. Thus, it should not automatically be assumed that the depressed child comes from a disturbed family.

What are some of the factors that seem to be associated with the development of depression? One of the most commonly cited problems is hostility and conflict in the home. It is not clear whether this hostility is directed toward the child in particular, or whether it is a more general problem that pervades the family or the marital relationship. Families with depressed children also tend to be inactive and uninvolved in either recreational, social, or intellectual/cultural activities. Thus, these youngsters do not have opportunities to experience pleasure, to develop psychosocially, to occupy their thoughts with something of a pleasant nature, or temporarily to escape from the family environment. A lack of emotional support and suppression of expression of any kind may also be present. The children may be given a minimum of say in decisions that affect them.

Although there have not been any large-scale studies of families with a depressed preschool-age child, which is in part a function of the fact that the disorder is relatively rare among children this young, it appears as though the families of such children are severely disturbed. The research conducted by Kashani and colleagues indicates that these families are characterized by extreme chaos, neglect, abuse, abuse of chemicals or alcohol, and psychopathology evident in a parent.

Results of the existing treatment outcome studies are encouraging and suggest that a variety of behavioral and cognitive techniques can be used effectively. A number of comprehensive treatment programs that combine behavioral and cognitive procedures have been developed. It appears as though these programs are effective in reducing the symptoms of depression. When the various literature bases are considered together, it appears as though the existing treatment programs need to be expanded to target the child's family as well as his or her classroom. Maladaptive family interactions that lead to and/ or maintain the youngster's depressogenic thinking and behavior need to be altered. In addition, steps need to be taken to ensure that the youngster receives short-term scholastic help to prevent school failures. Such a program will be described in the following chapters.

3

Implementation Issues in Treatment

IDENTIFICATION OF DEPRESSED CHILDREN

Depressed children can come to the school psychologist's attention through a variety of pathways. A child may be referred for a psychological evaluation through the traditional path of a teacher referral. A teacher might report that the child's academic performance has declined, the child seems unusually morose, cries frequently, is angry, withdrawn, or the child "has low self-esteem." School counselors are another major source of referrals. Their referrals often are similar in description to those made by teachers. Less frequently, a child's parents may refer their child for a psychological evaluation for many of the same reasons. Occasionally, a young adolescent will be referred by a classmate when the classmate becomes concerned about a friend's extreme withdrawal, dysphoric affect, or talk of suicide.

Even though schools have so many concerned individuals who serve as potential referral sources, the vast majority of depressed children are never identified. Steps have to be taken to improve the skills of the traditional referral agents, additional school personnel need to be included in the identification process, and the school psychologist has to take a more active role in the identification of depressed youths. The discussion now turns to steps that can be taken to increase the number of depressed children who are identified in the school.

Educating Referral Agents

Combating Misbeliefs

Depressed children are underidentified for a variety of reasons. One reason is that there are a number of commonly held beliefs in our society that preclude the existence of depression as a serious problem during childhood. Alerting potential referral agents to these misbeliefs is a first step toward educating these individuals. Perhaps the most common misbelief is that childhood is a carefree time of happiness. For many adults, this is true of their recollections of childhood. Those adults who did not have happy childhoods often do not admit it, and they consider themselves to be the unfortunate exception to the rule. Although this old adage may or may not have been true in the past, children today are growing up under much greater pressure, with less support at home, and in an increasingly impersonal and depersonalizing environment that involves a much more restricted range of interpersonal contact and activity.

Depression is often considered to be the result of, or reaction to, some traumatic or disappointing event. If no known tragedy has occurred, then how can the child be depressed? An unpleasant experience certainly is not the sole etiological factor in the development of depression. This assumption also includes the corollary misbelief that children are impacted by the same events that are associated with depression among adults. Because of developmental differences and differences in learning histories, events that would not faze an adult might be very distressing for a child. Additionally, a series of less apparent or dramatic events, rather than one major event, could, given the appropriate circumstances, trigger the onset of depression.

Depressive symptoms may be overlooked because of the belief that children go through phases, including moody phases, that they eventually outgrow. This belief fails to recognize the breadth, severity, and duration of the symptoms. It also fails to recognize the long-term impact of the disorder on the youngster's psychosocial functioning.

While consulting with a group of teachers from a local elementary school recently, I was struck by the degree of responsibility these teachers held for the welfare of their students. They truly felt as though they were responsible for trying to meet *all* of the needs of each child in their classrooms. Thus, if a child seemed "down," they felt it was their responsibility to cheer that child up. If the child seemed to have poor self-esteem, they felt it was their responsibility to devise a way to boost the youngster's self-esteem.

These teachers viewed a referral for a special education evaluation as a personal failure. They believed that such a referral meant that they were inadequate as teachers and had let that child down. As a result, they held off making referrals until they had tried everything they knew, or they did not make a referral so that they could try one more new idea. They were extremely conscientious and ingenious in their efforts. However, the depressed child would have been better served through an early referral for individual counseling combined with consultation to support and guide the teacher's efforts to help.

Perhaps the biggest reason that more children are not referred by their teachers is that depressed children rarely act out. Commonly, they are quiet children who sit in the back of the room and do not say much at all. When they are asked to do something, they usually are eager to please the teacher and very compliant. It is easy for these children to be forgotten. Unfortunately, the old adage that "the squeaky wheel gets the grease" applies here. Depressed children do not demand the attention of their teachers or other school personnel.

Direct Education

The referral agent may not recognize that a child is depressed because he or she is unfamiliar with how depression manifests itself during childhood. An in-service lesson for the school staff may help the relevant referral agents to recognize symptoms of depression. The school psychologist can use Chapter 1 of this book as a resource for developing descriptions of the symptoms of depression to present to the teachers and other school personnel. In addition, the psychologist may want to disseminate a copy of Bauer's (1987) article entitled "A Teacher's Introduction to Childhood Depression." This article provides the reader with a brief, easily understood, although basic, description of how depression may be exhibited in the classroom. A key part of this article is a table that lists the possible ways that depression can be manifested in the classroom. A revised edition of this table appears in Table 3.1.

Following the description of the symptoms of depression, it is very helpful to facilitate a discussion about how children express their depression. This enables the participants to ask questions. It also helps the staff learn to distinguish between depression and other psychological disorders. One of the phenomena we have observed after doing such in-services is that suddenly most of the referred children have a label of depression attached to them. Thus, a discussion that focuses on differentiating depression from other problems is important. In addition, it is important to provide the referral

TABLE 3.1. Possible Manifestations of Depression in the Classroom

Academic indicators

Unexplainable decline in school performance
Loss of interest in school subjects
Decline in effort expended
Work becomes messy or has an appearance that suggest that the child does not care how it looks
Child gives up easily
Child stops completing assigned work
Complains of not having enough energy to complete schoolwork

Social/behavioral indicators

Agitation/hyperactivity
Increased dependence
Regression to playing with younger children
Antisocial behavior (e.g., lying, stealing)
Bodily complaints
Disruptive classroom behavior
Phobias
Falls asleep during class
Looks and acts tired
Alienates peers
Unpopular
Withdraws from social contact

Cognitive indicators

Indecisiveness
Concentration difficulties
Expressions of suicidal wishes
Expects to do poorly/fail
Thoughts about death

Affective indicators

Poor self-esteem
Irritable
Complains excessively
Dysphoria
Feels guilty

Physical indicators

Sleep disturbance
Excessive weight gain or loss
Change in appetite
Feels weighted down
Psychomotor disturbance
Complains about feeling tired

Note. Adapted from Bauer (1987).

agents with some corrective feedback when it is ethically appropriate to do so as they refer youngsters to you for "depression."

Expanding the Referral Base

A number of other professionals in the school who can play an important role in the identification of depressed children are often overlooked in the special education referral process. At one of the middle schools where I regularly consult, the school nurse has been brought into the identification process. The school nurse is in an unique position to help in the identification of depressed children because depressed children frequent the nurse's office complaining about bodily concerns. The most common complaints are stomachaches and headaches. They also show up at the nurse's office complaining of fatigue and/or general physical malaise. The well-trained school nurse would also become concerned when he or she notices that a child has lost or gained an unusually large amount of weight. Another red flag is raised when a child maintains the same weight over an extended period of time while he or she is growing. The nurse also might notice, or be alerted to, some suspicious physical complaints or wounds that are suggestive of suicidal behavior. For example, the child may have scratches or cuts on the wrists, or the youngster may report being ill because of "accidently swallowing too many aspirin."

Administrators can be another important referral agent. They frequently have access to information to which no one else is privy. Since they are central figures in school to whom many people report, including people from the community, they often are the only ones who know a child's parents are having problems that might be stressful for their child. In addition, they frequently are contacted by law enforcement personnel when a child gets into trouble or runs away. Thus, they may have a more complete picture of a youngster than anyone else in the school. Administrators also are in an unique position because they are responsible for straightening out disagreements, investigating disciplinary complaints, and disciplining youngsters. In this role, they acquire a great deal of information. In addition, disciplinary meetings often are highly emotional situations in which the child reveals personal information that would not come out elsewhere. The sensitive and psychologically sophisticated administrator can pursue openings or leads that the child might give.

Greater support and involvement from parents in the community is very desirable. It would be helpful to educate a relatively large sample of parents about the nature of childhood depression and the extent of the problem. The traditional method of a school-sponsored evening with professionals who lecture briefly and answer questions is one way to convey information to groups of parents. However, this procedure often fails because the parents who are most in need of the information fail to attend. A clever principal in a local elementary school has developed a way to overcome this problem. His school combines a hot-dog and ice-cream social along with the panel of professionals who speak and address parental questions. To ensure attendance, and that the parents who most need the information receive it, he holds a contest in every classroom for complimentary tickets to the hot-dog and ice-cream dinner. The children are encouraged to enter their family's name into a box in each classroom. Each classroom teacher draws names from the box, and names of families that could really benefit from the information are added to the list of winners. The next day the names of the winners are announced, and free admission certificates are mailed home. Fliers announcing the evening are sent home with all children.

During the presentation to the parents, the psychologist describes the symptoms of depression, the impact of depression on social relationships and school performance, the prevalence of the problem; commonly held misbeliefs are dispelled, and the psychologist offers information about referral resources and school programs for depressed youngsters. Parents are encouraged to take action by referring their child for help if it appears as though he or she needs it. When describing depression and answering questions, it is important to keep in mind that parents often assume responsibility for their child's problems. Thus, a good deal of sensitivity to this issue needs to be kept in mind when speaking.

Even in school districts with enlightened staff, administrators, and parents, the vast majority of depressed children go unidentified. In fact, our research (Stark, Kendall, et al., 1990) indicates that fewer than 5% of the depressed children identified through the multiple-gate assessment process described below have been classified as emotionally disturbed. A need exists for school psychologists to take an active role in the identification of depressed children.

Multiple-Gate Assessment Model

Since 1980, a number of paper-and-pencil self-report measures of depression during childhood have appeared in the literature. These questionnaires consist of lists of the behavioral, cognitive, affective, physical, and motivational symptoms of depression. On some questionnaires such as the CDI (Kovacs, 1981), each symptom is described three times, with each description varying along a dimension of severity from normal to severe levels. The child is instructed to endorse the statement that best describes how the child has felt over the past 2 weeks. On other measures, such as the CDS (Reynolds, 1987b), each symptom is described. Following the description is a Likert-type rating scale that varies along a frequency dimension. The child is instructed to endorse the frequency rating that best describes how often he or she experienced the symptom over the past week. Since I have found the range of symptom ratings on the CDI to be too restricted and children to be unreliable reporters of the frequency of their depressive symptoms, I have developed the Child and Adolescent Depression Inventory. This measure includes four descriptions of the manifestation of each symptom of depression. An attempt has been made to include a more extreme expression of each symptom. This seems to help reduce the number of false positives, as children who are feeling dysphoria tend to be able to distinguish the more clinically relevant expressions from the normal feelings. Sample items from this measure are included in Figure 3.1.

A list of the self-report questionnaires that have appeared in the literature and their authors is provided in Table 3.2. There have been numerous review articles in the literature in which the psychometric properties of these measures have been described (see Kazdin, 1981; Kendall, Cantwell, & Kazdin, 1989; Kerr, Hoier, & Versi, 1987; Petti, 1978; Reynolds, 1984; Weller & Weller, 1985). In general, results of the psychometric investigations indicate that the self-report measures are reliable, and have adequate convergent validity, but lack discriminant validity. Because of their poor discriminant validity, it has been recommended that self-report measures only be used as screening devices (Stark, Kaslow, Hill, et al., 1990), whereas interviews should be used for diagnostic purposes as well as for determining the severity of the symptoms of depression.

A few clinical interviews have been developed for assessing depression and other childhood disorders, and these measures have adequate psychometric properties. Included among these measures are the Bellevue Index of Depression (Petti, 1978), Children's Depression Rating Scale — Revised (Poznanski et al., 1984), and the Schedule for Affective Disorders and Schizophrenia for School-Age Children (K-SADS; Puig-Antich & Ryan, 1986). Once again, the interested reader is referred to the aforementioned review articles for specific information about the psychometric properties of these instruments. Unlike the self-report measures, the interviews require some training to be administered in a reliable and valid fashion. Thus, their use is somewhat limited by the fact that few school

1. [   ] I feel happy.
   [   ] I feel OK.
   [   ] I feel sad.
   [   ] I feel so sad that it hurts.

3. [   ] I feel happy or OK.
   [   ] I'm sad, and I can be cheered up.
   [   ] I'm sad, and when you cheer me up, I go back to feeling sad.
   [   ] I'm sad, and nothing can cheer me up.

11. [   ] I haven't felt like crying.
    [   ] I know why I felt like crying.
    [   ] I know why I cried.
    [   ] I cried and I didn't even know why.

13. [   ] I do not think about killing myself.
    [   ] I have passing thoughts about killing myself, but I wouldn't.
    [   ] I have thought of specific ways to kill myself.
    [   ] I tried, or want to try, to kill myself.

14. [   ] I want to be by myself.
    [   ] Sometimes I avoid being with people.
    [   ] Being with people is OK.
    [   ] I like being with people.

FIGURE 3.1. Sample items from the Child and Adolescent Depression Inventory.

psychologists receive training in the administration of these measures. However, there are workshops being given around the country that include training on these interviews.

We have used the Present Episode Version of the K-SADS in the research being conducted through the Childhood Depression Project at The University of Texas. At this time, 243 children have been interviewed, and the results indicate that the K-SADS is internally consistent, has adequate interrater reliability, and that diagnoses can be reliably made based on the K-SADS interview.

The K-SADS interview yields a plethora of clinical information. It enables the interviewer to gather information about additional psychopathology that might co-occur with depression. This is important, since it is very common for additional disorders to co-occur with depression. In fact, depression occurs less frequently in isolation than it does in combination with other disorders.

The K-SADS includes questions that help the interviewer determine the time of onset of the current episode of depression as well as the duration of the episode. The interview assesses the presence and

TABLE 3.2. Self-Report Measures for Assessing Depression in Children and Their Authors

Title	Author
Children's Depression Inventory (7–17 years)	Kovacs (1981)
Child Depression Scale (8–13 years)	Reynolds (1987a, 1987b)
Children's Depression Scale (9–16 years)	Lang & Tisher (1978)
Child and Adolescent Depression Inventory (8–18 years)	Stark (1990)

severity of 21 symptoms of depression at two potentially different points in time: when the symptom was experienced at its most severe level over the past 12 months and how it was experienced over the past week. A list of the symptoms that are assessed with the K-SADS can be found in Table 3.3.

The K-SADS is a semistructured interview that requires 45 minutes to 1½ hours to complete. The interview manual provides the interviewer with a series of potential questions that serves as a guide. The interviewer chooses among the questions the ones that he or she believes will elicit the relevant information. Each symptom is assessed in depth. Perhaps it is because of this level of detail and specificity that we have found that children often reveal information for the first time during the K-SADS interview. For example, a number of children have disclosed for the first time that they have been victims of abuse.

Interviewing depressed children can be a challenge. Often, be-

TABLE 3.3. List of the Symptoms of Depression That Can Be Assessed with the K-SADS

1. Dysphoric mood	12. Psychomotor retardation
2. Angry/irritable feelings	13. Social withdrawal
3. Excessive guilt	14. Anhedonia
4. Feeling unloved	15. Sleep disturbance
5. Self-esteem	16. Hypersomnia
6. Self-pity	17. Anorexia
7. Somatic complaints	18. Overeating
8. Worries about health	19. Self-damage
9. Fatigue	20. Suicidal ideation
10. Difficulty concentrating	21. Suicidal behavior
11. Psychomotor agitation	

cause of the various symptoms of depression, they are very withdrawn and quiet. They spontaneously offer very little information. Rather, the information has to be drawn out of them. Their answers are short, frequently "yes," "no" responses. Thus, in order to obtain the desired information, the interviewer has to work very hard. Typically, these youngsters do not respond well to open-ended questions since their answers are short and do not supply the desired information. As a result of these limitations, a more structured approach is necessary when interviewing depressed children.

The sample interview provided in Appendix A illustrates some of these points. First, the interviewer asks very specific questions that can be answered with minimal responses. Each question and answer in isolation provide the interviewer with a small piece of information, and when all of the questions and answers are considered simultaneously, a big picture emerges. The interview is semistructured. Thus, there is a goal-directed reason for almost all of the questions. The goal is the identification of depressive symptoms and the measurement of the severity of these symptoms. By being so focused, it also reduces the amount of time needed to acquire the information. The questions use concrete anchors to help the children answer questions that require fine-grained discriminations (e.g., Do you feel sad from the time you awaken until the time you eat lunch?). As a whole, the interview seems somewhat leading, but this results from the differences in technique required for successfully interviewing a depressed child.

Because of the limitations in the discriminant validity of the paper-and-pencil self-report measures of depression and the time-consuming nature of the interviews, a multiple-gate assessment procedure has been developed (e.g., Reynolds, 1986) that makes maximum use of the advantages of both types of assessment procedures. The process is outlined in Figure 3.2 and is designed to reduce the number of false positives (children who indicate that they are depressed on a paper-and-pencil measure when in fact they are not depressed) that are interviewed. As can be seen in Figure 3.2, a self-report measure such as the CDI is used as a screening device. It is completed by large numbers of children in large groups, such as entire classrooms of children. The measures are scored, and all of those children who score above the suggested cut-off score of 19 (Kovacs, 1983) go on to the next stage of the process. The children who score less than 19 discontinue the process and are considered not to be depressed. A second determining factor in what is done with a child is the youngster's response to the suicide question. If the

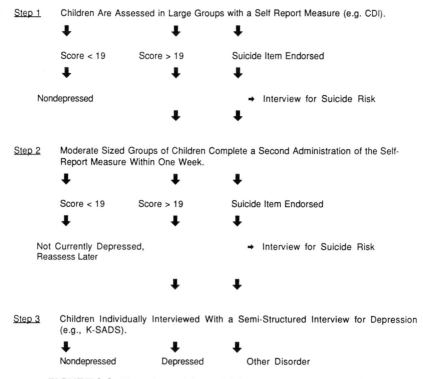

FIGURE 3.2. Flow chart of the multiple-gate assessment procedure.

youngster endorses the statement "I want to kill myself," he or she is immediately interviewed to determine the possibility of suicidal risk.

The children who scored 19 or greater on the first administration of the CDI complete a second administration within 1 week of the first test. Those children who once again score less than 19 and do not indicate any suicidal intent are considered not to be depressed. They may be reassessed in the future. The youngsters who indicate suicidal intent are interviewed for suicidal risk, and the children who once again score a 19 or greater progress on to the third phase.

During the third phase, the children are interviewed with an instrument such as the K-SADS. Although this is a lengthy process, it saves a lot of the therapist's time because it greatly reduces the number of children who have to be interviewed. For example, in 1988, 720 children completed an initial administration of the CDI as part of the Childhood Depression Project. One hundred and sixteen scored a 19 or greater on the first CDI. Seventy-seven of the 104 children who received parental permission and completed a second administration of the CDI scored 19 or greater. Thus, by using two administrations of the CDI, the number of children who needed to be interviewed was reduced by 39 (37.5%), thus reducing the number of hours spent interviewing children by 40 to 60 hours. As a result of the K-SADS interview, 33 (43%) children received a diagnosis of a depressive disorder. Thus, even after taking these steps, the vast majority of the children who scored above the cut-off score on the CDI were not seriously depressed.

ASSESSMENT-GUIDED INTERVENTION

As noted above, the K-SADS provides the therapist with a great deal of information. This information can also be used to guide treatment. The therapist can review the results of the interview and identify the problematic symptoms. For example, the child may report sleep disturbance that would then become a target of change. The therapist would use certain behavioral (e.g., relaxation training) and cognitive (e.g., imagery, distraction) techniques to reduce the severity of the sleep disturbance. Although the K-SADS and CDI give the examiner a great deal of information, they don't make up the complete picture. Additional assessment is necessary.

The assessment process begins by the therapist's trying to answer a couple of very basic questions. The first is: At what level should I intervene? Should I work directly with the child? Do I need to intervene with the youngster's family or at some other environmental level? Commonly, it is necessary to intervene at both (child and family/environmental) of these levels. Nevertheless, at each of these two levels, more specific assessment questions need to be addressed. When assessing the child, some of the corollary questions are: Is the child experiencing a cognitive disturbance, and if so, does it take the form of a deficit or distortion in thinking? What are the child's expectations for the future, and how does the child attribute causality? Is the child experiencing a behavioral skills deficit? If so, is the disturbance the result of a cognitive impairment or a skills deficit. If it does result from a skills deficit, what is the nature of the deficit? Does the child need social skills or assertiveness skills training? What specific skills is the child deficient in? Is the child experiencing a deficit in self-control skills? For example, is the child self-monitoring negative events to the exclusion of positive events?

To answer the previous questions, a variety of tools can be used. A number of additional procedures for assessing cognitions are discussed in Chapter 4. In addition to these procedures, the school psychologist might want to use some of the tools noted in Table 3.4. Procedures and questionnaires that can be used to assess behavioral and self-control skills are listed in this table.

The other primary area that needs to be assessed is the child's

TABLE 3.4. Assessment Tools That Can Be Used to Complete a Thorough Cognitive-Behavioral Assessment of Depression

Target of treatment	Possible assessment tools
Cognitive disturbance	
Deficit	Matching Familiar Figures Test (Kagan, Rosman, Day, Albert, & Phillips, 1964)
Distortion	Cognitive Triad Inventory for Children (CTI-C; Kaslow et al., 1990)
	Automatic Thoughts Questionnaire for Children (Stark, Best, & McCabe, 1990)
	Cognitive Bias Questionnaire for Children (Haley, Fine, Marriage, Morretti, & Freeman, 1985)
	Projectives (e.g., CAT or TAT, Rorschach, drawings)
Negative expectancies for the future	Hopelessness Scale for Children (Kazdin et al., 1983)
Self-control deficits	
Self-monitoring	Pleasant and Unpleasant Events Schedules for Children
	Automatic Thoughts Questionnaire for Children (Stark et al., 1987)
	Projectives such as TATs
Self-evaluation	My Standards Questionnaire—Revised (Stark, Adam, & Best, 1986)
	Self-Esteem Inventory (Coopersmith, 1967)
Self-reward	(see Kaslow et al., 1984)
Behavioral deficits	
Social skills	Matson Evaluation of Social Skills for Youths (Matson, Rotatori, & Helsel, 1983)
	Observation of free play
Assertiveness skills	Observation of social interactions
Related pathology	
Anxiety	Projectives
	Children's Manifest Anxiety Scale—Revised (Reynolds & Richmond, 1985)

home environment and his or her family relationships and interactions. This assessment is guided by the following question: What is happening, or has happened, that has led to and is currently maintaining the disturbance in the child's thinking and behavior? The patterns of interaction, messages about the child, the world, and the future being communicated, the disciplinary methods of the parents, maladaptive family rules, and the structural characteristics of the family are assessed. The primary means of assessing these variables is through joining the family and observing their interactions. No single measure or combination of measures has been developed for assessing all of these variables. The disturbed patterns that are likely to be found among families with depressed children have been described elsewhere (Stark & Brookman, in press).

The important point to be made here is that assessment is used as a guide to treatment. Once assessment reveals a disturbance in a given area, then this area becomes a target for intervention. It also is important to note that, in keeping with the behavioral tradition, assessment is an ongoing process. It is continually used to guide (see below) and evaluate treatment. When it is used to evaluate treatment effectiveness, the severity of depressive symptomatology is assessed every other session. In the adult literature (e.g., Rehm et al., 1987) severity of depression is commonly assessed with a self-report measure (e.g., BDI; Beck et al., 1961) every session. However, we have found this to be too time-consuming and tedious for children. Thus, we have developed a symptom checklist (see Appendix B) that can be completed with a minimum of effort in a few minutes. The children simply indicate the presence or absence of each symptom.

SELECTION OF TREATMENT PROCEDURES

When conducting research, we have combined the treatment procedures into a package in which the participants are taught one skill or technique and then the next in a logical, additive sequence. This sequence and the time frame for delivery are presented in Table 3.5. In addition, the goals and subgoals for each session are outlined in Appendix C. This outline is specific enough to provide the reader with a guide to implementing a packaged treatment program. This preset, programmatic approach to the delivery of treatment is a reflection both of the need to create methodological rigor in our research and of the fact that a multicomponent treatment program is required for most depressed children. When working with individuals in clinical practice, we are more flexible and choose from the

TABLE 3.5. Timeline and Sequence of Training Procedures Used in Stark et al. (1989)

Week 1

Session 1   Introductions, discuss confidentiality, complete a group activity, discussion of participants' perceptions of treatment

Session 2   Introduction to treatment rationale, complete a group activity

Week 2

Session 3   Review and extend treatment rationale, complete a group activity

Session 4   Review and extend treatment rationale, complete a group activity

Week 3

Session 5   Review treatment rationale and begin training in self-reinforcement

Session 6   Review and extend training in self-reinforcement

Week 4

Session 7   Review and extend training in self-reinforcement

Session 8   Review and extend training in self-reinforcement

Week 5

Session 9   Review self-reinforcement, begin training in self-monitoring of pleasant events

Session 10   Review self-monitoring of pleasant events and add activity scheduling

Week 6

Session 11   Review self-monitoring and activity scheduling

Session 12   Review activity scheduling and introduce relaxation training

Week 7

Session 13   Review and begin assertiveness training

Session 14   Assertiveness training

Week 8

Session 15   Assertiveness training

Session 16   Social skills training

Week 9

Session 17   Social skills training

Week 10

Session 18   Social skills training

Week 11

Session 19   Review and make social skills video

(continued)

TABLE 3.5. (cont.)

Week 12	
Session 20	Introduction to cognitive restructuring and personal scientist approach (begin use of thought records)
Week 13	
Session 21	Review and extension of cognitive restructuring
Week 14	
Session 22	Review and introduction to problem solving
Week 15	
Session 23	Problem-solving mastery exercises
Week 16	
Session 24	Attribution training
Week 17	
Session 25	Self-evaluation training
Week 18	
Session 26	Working toward self-improvement
All subsequent sessions	Continued work toward self-improvement using all of the previously learned skills

myriad of procedures presented below those that are most relevant to each child. It is not an efficient use of time to work in areas where there are no problems. Why teach social skills to a socially adept child? The selection of treatment procedures is guided by the results of a thorough cognitive and behavioral assessment that was presented in Table 3.4. Since assessment is an ongoing process, the choice of treatment procedures may change as new information is gathered and synthesized. We also are more flexible in the timing of the presentation of the treatment procedures. With more severely impaired youngsters, we begin with a behavioral approach that is designed to secure more immediate symptom relief. This helps the child to attain some distance from, and control over, his or her thinking and the associated negative emotions.

As indicated in Table 3.4, there are a number of assessment devices at this time that can be used to guide the selection of treatment procedures. If a youngster indicates difficulty in the area being assessed, then use of the corresponding treatment procedure is indicated. For example, if a distortion in thinking is indicated on the CTI-C, then cognitive restructuring procedures would be indicated.

Likewise, if the child reported an adaptive attributional style, then attribution retraining would not be utilized.

In general, across children the core components of the treatment program seem to remain the same. This core includes cognitive restructuring, training in self-control skills, and parent-training/family therapy. Most of the flexibility appears to be in choosing the specific cognitive procedures and in the use of the behavioral procedures.

If a number of depressed children have been identified, necessitating the formation of groups, then each child's specific problem areas are identified through the assessment process, and groups are formed according to similarities in clinical picture. Since the core components of treatment typically are the same, it is relatively easy to implement the treatment program in groups. Usually this means that some children will receive some remediation in areas that are not deficient. This does not seem to be of any harm, and time saved through group administration outweighs time spent working in areas where any one child is not deficient. In addition, this seems to allow these children to shine as they can show off their skills and knowledge. These skillful youngsters should be encouraged to act as collaborative tutors for their less skilled peers.

THERAPEUTIC HOMEWORK

As implied in the previous sections that describe the treatment procedures, therapeutic homework is a key ingredient of the treatment program. The child spends only 45 minutes to 2 hours a week in direct contact with the therapist or treatment group. When this is considered in the light of the severity of the problem and the complexity of the treatment program, this represents a very small portion of the youngster's week. Furthermore, since the goal of treatment is the acquisition of coping skills, it is imperative to maximize the amount of time the child spends working on mastering the skills. One way to overcome these obstacles and to accomplish these objectives is to get the child working outside of treatment as well as in the sessions. Therapeutic homework can be used to do this.

Children typically are turned off by the thought of having to do homework. Thus, one basic rule that I follow is to never refer to it as "homework." The term "practice" is used instead. Most children are at least somewhat resistant to doing homework. This is even more of a problem with depressed youngsters. On top of the normal youthful dislike of homework, the depressed child has a number of symptoms that exacerbate this. For example, because of fatigue the child may not feel as though he or she has the energy to do the homework. Similarly, because of difficulty concentrating, the child may lose track of what he or she is supposed to be doing. The youngster's pessimism and anhedonia especially are problematic, since they lead the child to believe that there is no reason to bother doing the homework because it is boring and will not help anyway. Thus, a number of special steps have to be taken to ensure that the depressed child completes his or her therapeutic homework.

First, whenever a homework assignment is given, the therapist has to be sure to talk about the outcome of the assignment at the start of the next session. This provides the child with some reinforcement for his or her efforts. Failing to talk about it is analogous to placing it on an extinction schedule. Since it is difficult for the child to complete all of the assignments, and this failure could have a countertherapeutic impact (e.g., confirm the belief that he can not do anything), it is important that the therapist maximizes the child's opportunity to be successful. In addition, emphasis should be placed on the youngster's efforts. In other words, trying to do it is praiseworthy in and of itself.

After giving a homework assignment, it is good practice to ask the child to repeat the assignment back to the therapist. This serves as a check of the youngster's understanding of the instructions. If the child does not understand what he or she has been asked to do, then the therapist re-explains the assignment. After the assignment has been given and the instructions are understood, the child is asked to write down the practice assignment on a sheet of paper. This paper is kept in a folder that the child carries to and from school on a daily basis. The child can refer to it whenever needed.

Another useful procedure is to ask the child to close his or her eyes and cognitively rehearse the assignment through imaging it. As the child images it, or immediately thereafter, the child can be instructed to identify potential impediments to completing the assignment successfully. If an impediment is identified, problem solving is used to develop a plan for overcoming the impediment. If it seems as though things are going too smoothly, then the therapist might pose some possible impediments and help the child develop plans for overcoming them.

When first giving the assignment, it is helpful to involve the child in the formulation of it. For example, a problem can be posed, and the child and therapist collaborate to develop a solution through a homework assignment. The child is helped to understand the rationale for the assignment and how it will help him or her overcome the problem. This understanding and participation go a long way toward ensuring that the child will complete his or her therapeutic homework.

Some depressed children require additional incentives that are externally administered. With these children, externally administered rewards can be used as incentives. A contract can be written that states that if the child completes his or her practice assignments, then the therapist will reward the child.

TIME FRAME

In a related vein, the time frame reported in Table 3.5 was utilized for research purposes and reflected the practical constraints of that specific situation. The actual time frame utilized for treatment should be guided by the client's response to it. Obviously children respond differently for a multitude of reasons; thus, the duration of treatment should be altered depending on each youngster's response. Given the ambitious goal of producing long-lasting, philosophical change, we recommend working with a child until he or she demonstrates an adaptive level of symptomatology *and* the ability to independently select and use the skills and techniques to control depressive symptoms. We have found that a semester or more may be required to accomplish this goal.

The spacing of the sessions should change over the course of treatment. In the beginning, and for the first month to 8 weeks, we recommend scheduling twice-weekly sessions. This helps to produce more rapid symptom control and relief. Subsequently, weekly sessions are scheduled until the youngster can start to self-modify his or her symptoms. At this point, sessions are scheduled biweekly, or on an as-needed basis until termination.

STRUCTURE OF SESSIONS

A fairly consistent pattern is evident in the use of time during each meeting. The beginning of each session is spent reviewing homework, and the last 5 to 10 minutes is spent assigning homework. Approximately half of the remaining time is spent talking about the clients' concerns, and the other half is spent in skills training. The actual mix of time varies dependent on the child and the point in treatment. Commonly, more time is spent eliciting client concerns in the beginning of treatment as rapport is being built. Then, there is a shift to more time being spent on skills building. Then, the mix varies primarily dependent on the child. If he or she is a fast learner and very open, then more time is spent discussing how he or she can apply the skills to his or her concerns. During the initial sessions of group treatment, the children usually are reluctant to bring up their personal concerns. Thus, this time is spent completing activities that are designed to produce trust and a sense of group cohesion (see "Affective Education" in Chapter 4). Once this is accomplished, the youngsters are more willing to disclose emotionally laden material.

THERAPISTS

To date, individuals with a wide variety of educational and professional experiences have served as the therapists in our empirically evaluated treatment endeavors, including graduate students in school and counseling psychology and clinical psychologists with years of experience. Highly structured therapists' manuals have been constructed in an attempt to guide the novice psychologists. However, it is not believed that someone without an understanding of cognitive–behavioral techniques who mechanically followed the treatment manuals could employ the treatment program in a maximally effective way. In fact, one of the most common mistakes made by students who implement the intervention program for the first time is that they rigidly follow the manual and fail to make it relevant to the children by tying it into the children's everyday problems. To maximize the effectiveness of the treatment program, it is important for the school psychologist to have an understanding of childhood depression as well as behavioral and cognitive–behavioral interventions.

DEVELOPMENTAL CONSIDERATIONS

Many of the concepts that are taught to the youngsters over the course of treatment are rather complex for a child to grasp. Thus, it is necessary to make the concepts more concrete and tied to their problems. Additionally, children find a didactic approach to teaching this information to be *boring*. Consequently, they lose interest in treatment very quickly if steps are not taken to make the treatment program understandable and engaging. A number of steps have been taken to accomplish this. Nonetheless, these may be the areas that will require the most work on the reader's part as he or she tries to implement the program.

We have relied heavily on the use of stories, cartoons, activities, and role playing to make the concepts more concrete and to present them in a more engaging fashion.

Story telling has proven to be one of the most reliable of these procedures. The youngsters easily relate to the stories and readily remember them. Many of the stories that are used describe the experience of youngsters who have participated in the treatment program over the years. An advantage of story telling is that the story can be individualized to fit the specific needs of the child. Stories can be created that help the child acquire and use the coping skills. They also help the child understand when he or she might use a particular skill, or how he or she might overcome an obstacle when trying to use a skill. Furthermore, the stories convey a sense of hope, since the child can see how other youngsters have improved as a result of treatment. For example, the following story has been particularly effective:

There was a girl I worked with who worked really hard the way you have. I want to tell you a story about this student that I knew a couple years ago. I'll call her Nicki since it wouldn't be right to use her real name. That would break our rule about confidentiality. She was in a group of sixth graders I was meeting with. When she came to the first meeting, she looked real down in the dumps. She never smiled and wore her hair over her eyes so no one could really see her. She didn't feel good about herself because she thought she wasn't pretty enough, she wasn't smart enough, and she felt she couldn't make friends. She'd look at the other kids and would think, "I'm not as good as them." During our meetings she hardly said a word. She didn't believe that anything could help her. So the first time I asked her to do some work at home, she reluctantly did it. She complained that it was too much work, and she'd rather just sit around and do nothing. But she did it, and she always listened to what everyone said in the group. She started to talk more and told the group about her family. She lived with her mom because her mom and dad had just gotten a divorce. Nicki thought that she had caused it, even though she really hadn't. Her mom always told her to do this and that. When she did these things, it was never good enough for her mom, so her mom would complain and punish Nicki. So Nicki was always getting grounded and scolded, which made her feel very down and worthless.

She felt tired a lot so she just sat around rather than playing with other kids. When other kids came over and asked her to play, she would tell them she couldn't — even when she could. Since she didn't feel good about herself, when she would play with other kids, she would only play with her younger sister's friends.

Since she wasn't very happy with her life, she listened very hard in our meetings and always did her practice exercises. With each passing meeting, she looked better and better. She got her hair cut so that you could see that she actually was pretty. She talked more and more and eventually started goofing around with the other kids. She started going out and playing with other kids her own age. She learned to identify the thoughts that made her feel sad, and she learned new, more realistic ones. She learned that she didn't have to be perfect, she didn't have to look like a model to be attractive, and she didn't have to be liked by everyone to be a good person. She started to like herself, and she learned how to talk to her mother so that she wouldn't always complain and tell her to do this and that.

A number of additional considerations should be kept in mind as the therapist is developing the stories. The characteristics of the main character of the story should be similar to those of the child. For example, the main character in the story would be the same gender, age, grade, and so forth, as the child client. In addition, the problems the child client has carrying out the treatment program would be incorporated into the story. The story character faces the problems and then overcomes them; thus, a coping model is used.

After telling the story, the major points of the story can be reviewed. Questions can be asked to determine whether the child has grasped the primary points of the story. If not, then the information can be reviewed. Additionally, the similarities between the child and the main character in the story can be discussed and related to the child.

Cartoon characters have been developed and arranged into short vignettes that illustrate a therapeutic concept or how to use the coping skills. For example, the cartoons in Figure 3.3 illustrate the use of self-monitoring. A variety of these cartoon sequences have been developed. They are compiled in a booklet that the child keeps. Oftentimes, parents report that their child has shown them the cartoons and explained the concept that was being illustrated. Some children color in the cartoons and add new thought bubbles. This outside use of the cartoons facilitates treatment generalization.

There are some additional cartoons that only include one picture. These cartoons are used as reminders by the children to use a coping skill or to complete therapeutic homework. For example, the children are instructed to place the cartoon in Figure 3.4 in readily noticeable places around the house such as in their bedrooms, on

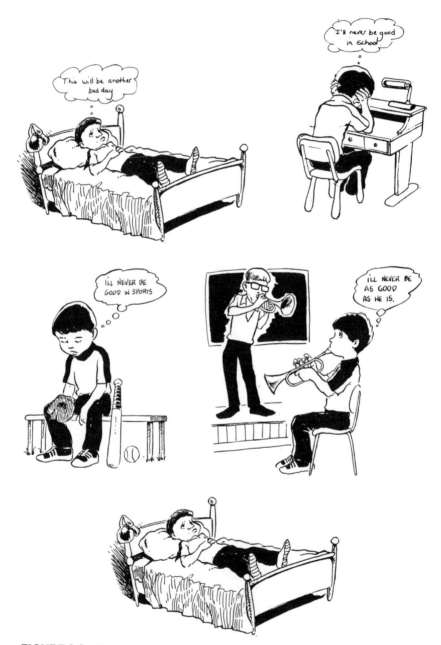

FIGURE 3.3. Cartoon sequence that illustrates the use of self-monitoring of cognitions.

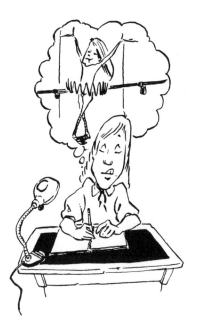

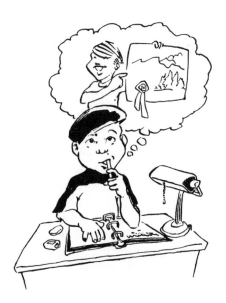

FIGURE 3.4. Homework reminder cartoons.

the desk or on the mirror. Likewise, the child might place a copy on the refrigerator. So that the child does not habituate to the cartoon, the therapist occasionally suggests that the child move it to new places.

Results of a questionnaire that has been given to treatment participants suggest that the cartoons had a positive impact on the participants. They helped the children remember what was discussed in the sessions. The children reported referring to the cartoons outside of the sessions. They also reported that the cartoons helped them to understand the concepts being taught.

THE THERAPEUTIC RELATIONSHIP

Importance of the Therapeutic Relationship

Numerous misperceptions exist about the nature of cognitive-behavior therapy. Perhaps one of the most common is that cognitive-behavior therapists are more concerned with technique than with the relationship they have with their clients. As a result of this misperception, it is often believed that cognitive–behavior therapists implement therapeutic techniques in a clinical and mechanical manner. Although it is true that cognitive–behavior therapists are more concerned with technique than are client-centered or humanistic therapists, they also recognize that the techniques are administered within the context of the client–therapist relationship (Goldfried & Davison, 1976). A solid client–therapist relationship is a prerequisite for the effective implementation of the treatment program described in the following chapters.

What are the characteristics of a good therapeutic relationship? It is a relationship that is characterized by mutual warmth, trust, and open and balanced communication, and a safe emotionally charged setting exists that culminates in an environment that enables the therapist to develop an empathic understanding of the child. Warmth is an affective characteristic of the relationship. It is a soft, positive emotional sensation. Trust refers to a belief that the other person does not want anything from you and that he or she will not do anything to harm you. Although a balance in communication is sought, the balance is not equal; rather, ideally, the client does more of the conversing. Both the client and the therapist determine the content of the sessions. Recognizing and addressing the client's current concerns is critical. Likewise, the therapist has a specific agenda that he or she is following, which keeps therapy progressing in a logical, focused, and change-producing direction.

There are two aspects to the last characteristic of the therapeutic relationship noted above. The interactions take place in an environment that is (1) safe and (2) emotionally charged. Safety is the perception of being secure from any threats of danger, harm, or personal loss. This sense of safety is fostered by the setting and the actions the therapist takes to ensure confidentiality. It also stems from the therapist's verbal behavior, whereby the child feels as though he or she is not being judged or evaluated by the therapist. It is a place to which the child can come and verbalize concerns, beliefs, emotional reactions, and so forth (within appropriate bounds) and not receive any negative consequences as a result of what is expressed. At times the therapeutic environment is emotionally charged. With depressed children, there is a tendency for the sessions to become dominated by unpleasant emotions; either sadness or anger, although some youngsters are devoid of affect, which produces a kind of hollow sense within the sessions. One of the goals of each session is to give the youngster an opportunity to experience a range of emotions, not just unpleasant emotions. In fact, some clinicians believe that it is essential for the depressed client to experience positive emotions during therapy sessions for therapy to have a long-term impact. As a result of sharing an emotional experience, whether it is primarily positive or negative, the bond between the child and therapist is strengthened.

Perhaps the most important characteristic of the therapeutic relationship is that the therapist develops an empathic understanding of the client. An empathic understanding is one in which the therapist has a deep understanding of the client's feelings, thoughts, and beliefs; and the therapist helps the client to gain a deeper understanding of his or her (the client's) thoughts, feelings, and actions. The therapist's goal is to be able to perceive the world through the client's eyes. This objective can hardly be emphasized enough. As noted later, an empathic understanding greatly facilitates cognitive restructuring. In fact, it seems as though gaining such an understanding of the client is a prerequisite for using cognitive restructuring procedures effectively.

A positive client–therapist relationship has a substantial therapeutic impact in and of itself. The relationship sends a number of important messages to the child that can lead to, or facilitate, change. First, it sends the message to the child that he or she is an important, worthwhile person who is likable even when he or she is having serious problems. This message contributes to a positive sense of self. Secondly, the collaborative nature of the relationship sends the youngster the message that he or she can manage his or her problems. This message contributes to a sense of self-efficacy.

Methods for Enhancing the Therapeutic Relationship

Collaboration

A distinct characteristic of the therapeutic relationship within the cognitive–behavioral perspective is collaboration. The client and therapist work *together* to solve the client's emotional upset and problems. The therapist works in an open manner with the client where he or she is fully informed about what is being done and why it is being done. The client plays an active and informed role in the treatment process, often directing the focus of intervention, independently gathering relevant information, and independently applying the therapeutic procedures. Of course this has to be done in a fashion that acknowledges the child's developmental level.

Therapist Considerations

The client–therapist relationship is enhanced by the perception that the therapist truly cares about the welfare of the youngster. This perception of caring is promoted directly and indirectly. The therapist, when appropriate, can tell the youngster in a sincere fashion that he or she cares about the child's welfare. In addition, this message of caring can be conveyed indirectly through the therapist's actions including being on time to sessions, not missing sessions, and taking additional actions that are designed to improve the child's life situation and depressive symptoms.

Another important consideration is the credibility of the therapist. Does the therapist project a sense of personal confidence and confidence in his or her therapeutic procedures? By virtue of the fact that the therapist is an adult in the role of a helper, and since adults are powerful people in a child's life, the therapist usually is automatically afforded some credibility. However, the projection of an attitude of confidence in one's own skills and in the therapeutic procedures that are being used enhances the therapist's credibility.

There are some things outside of the therapist's own actions that might undermine his or her credibility. One of the youngster's peers may tell the child that he or she saw a psychologist/counselor and "he didn't help at all." Similarly, a peer might report that she saw a psychologist and "he always sided with my parents and told my parents everything I said about them." The child's parents also are a potential source of counterproductive information that might undermine the therapist's credibility. The parents might call the therapist a "shrink" or "quack." In one instance, a parent told the child that the therapist was just "watching out for the school's interest and not yours." A parent also might openly question the value of going to therapy: "It's all a sham. He really can't do anything to help you."

The most effective way to promote a sense of credibility is to help produce positive change in the child's symptoms or life situation. To this end, it is a useful practice initially to choose a target of change that is readily, or at least more easily, changed. Nothing works like success to create a sense of credibility. This is especially critical for depressed youngsters who also are feeling hopeless.

Additional Methods

There are a number of additional methods that the therapist can employ to enhance the therapeutic relationship. One of the simplest procedures is to keep logs of important information about each child. Information such as names of siblings, birth date, parent's occupations, favorite shows, favorite recreational activities, best friends' names, and so forth is recorded in the log and reviewed by the therapist from time to time. At opportune times, the therapist uses the information to make comments that demonstrate to the child that he or she cares enough about him or her to remember such information. This helps the child feel special and as though the therapist really cares.

The therapist also conveys a sense of caring or concern through his or her nonverbal behavior. The therapist demonstrates that he or she cares by listening intently, giving the child eye contact, keeping an appropriate distance, and, at appropriate times, giving the youngster a pat on the back, shoulder, or elbow.

The therapist's demeanor during the sessions has an impact on the therapeutic relationship. It is important for the therapist to be pleasant and to display a sense of humor. Maintaining a sense of humor is especially important for working with depressed youths. Humor can be used as a gauge of how severely depressed the child client is. It also can be used to reduce the intensity of a session or to take the edge off a confrontation. In addition, it makes the sessions more enjoyable. Humor during the sessions results in the sharing of a positive emotional experience that strengthens the client–therapist relationship.

One of the primary foci of cognitive–behavioral therapy is the child-client's thoughts and beliefs. This includes the child's thoughts and beliefs about the therapeutic process and the therapist. The therapist openly and directly elicits the client's thoughts about therapy and the therapist. The therapist asks the child at the end of each session whether there was anything that he or she said or did during the session that bothered him or her (Beck, Rush, Shaw, & Emery, 1979). These are especially important questions to ask of the depressed child, since he or she is likely to distort the therapist's comments and actions in a negative way. Thus, something the therapist says or does can be misconstrued as a personal affront. Likewise, it is important to openly and directly discuss the youngster's thoughts about the therapeutic process. The child may have unrealistic expectations about change. Or the child might simply misunderstand why something is being done.

Unique Aspects of Depressed Youths

There are a number of unique characteristics of depressed children that can impact the therapeutic relationship. First, their depressed mood is an impediment. It drains the therapist's energy and can be contagious. Some of the doctoral students I have supervised have reported feeling quite depressed after spending an hour with a depressed child. The child often has a very distressing story to tell. It is easy to get caught up in the youngster's pessimism and discouraging situation. This is highly counterproductive. It is important for the therapist to acknowledge the youngster's perceptions of his or her life situation. However, it is equally important for the therapist to remember that depressed youngsters have a tendency to see things in a hopeless and unrealistically negative manner. Furthermore, it is important for the therapist to approach the things that are upsetting the child as problems to be solved just like any other problems. This helps both the client and therapist to take a more objective view of what is happening. Furthermore, it counters the sense of hopelessness.

The anhedonic depressed child creates special problems. He or she is bored much of the time, as he or she does not derive normal levels of pleasure from things, and the breadth of pleasurable events is reduced. The anhedonic youngster seems just to go through the motions of treatment. The child does not seem engaged in treatment. As a result of the youngster's bland affect, he or she also does not provide the therapist with much rewarding feedback. The child does not seem to be enjoying therapy. In fact, the child is likely to complain about having to do too much work, or that he or she is not having any fun. Treatment is "boring." This may be more of a reflection of the child's anhedonia than of a poor treatment plan. Nonetheless, the anhedonic youngster is more demanding of the therapist's patience, creativity, and ability to engage the child.

Depressed youngsters are hopeless. This hopelessness can lead to a sense of frustration in the therapist. The child at times seems unwilling to follow the therapist's suggestions or to take actions to improve his or her plight. The solution to a situation or the action to take to feel better may have been made perfectly clear to the child by the therapist, yet the depressed youngster does nothing or acts in a countertherapeutic way. Some practicum students have noted that they felt like telling the child to "wake-up," or like shaking the youngster into taking action. Needless to say, this interferes with the development of a positive bond between the therapist and client.

Working within the school creates some additional unique roadblocks to the establishment of a good therapeutic relationship. First, adults who work in schools are generally lumped by children into the same category: authoritarian figures who can potentially punish the students. From this perspective, it is not clear how much the therapist can be trusted. The youngster is concerned that he or she may say something wrong or reveal something that could lead to punishment. Concerns about confidentiality are much greater. Students worry about whether their peers or teachers are going to hear about what they have talked about. In addition, they often are quite sensitive about their classmates and teachers knowing that they are seeing the school psychologist. Thus, there are some additional strains on the client–therapist relationship in the school that the therapist needs to be aware of and to address directly through inquiry.

REFERRAL CONSIDERATIONS

When treating depressed children, it is important to consider the severity of the disorder and the therapist's skills, and it is important to set aside any biases or preconceived notions about psychiatric consultation. If the child is severely depressed, chronically depressed, or potentially suicidal, it is in the child's best interests to consult with a psychiatrist. If the child is actively suicidal, then a referral for hospitalization is necessary. Thus, if the child is diagnosed as expriencing major depression or a long-standing dysthymic disorder, then a psychiatric consultation is warranted. Descriptions of ways to gauge the severity of each symptom were offered in Chapter 1.

Another consideration that enters into the severity formula is the nature of the child's home life. Does the child come from a healthy, functional, and supportive family; or does she come from a psychologically abusive, chaotic, hostile, and nonsupportive family? The more destructive the family situation, the more likely that temporary removal in the form of hospitalization will facilitate positive change. It also might serve as the crisis that pushes the family to seek treatment. Most of the better hospital programs for psychologically disturbed youngsters include an intense family therapy component.

The treatment package described in this book is a complex one that necessitates an understanding of the cognitive–behavioral perspective. Since some of the procedures described in Chapters 4 and 5 may be new to the reader, it is recommended that supervision be sought from a psychologist with experience in cognitive–behavioral therapy. Workshops and additional course work at a university also may be helpful. Another personal consideration is the amount of experience the therapist has with depressed children. Since depressed youths pose a number of unique problems for the therapist, it is important to acquire additional information about depressed children. This book serves as one step in this process. Additional reading and supervised experience are helpful. Finally, the therapist should consider how working with depressed children will impact the therapist on a personal level. Depressed children can have a depressing impact on the therapist. It is important to maintain an awareness of the youngster's impact.

A pragmatic consideration in making a referral decision is the amount of time that the school psychologist has for working with the depressed youngster. The comprehensive treatment program described in this book is quite demanding of the psychologist's time. The therapist has to be prepared for twice-weekly sessions for a 2- to 8-week period and weekly sessions for at least an additional 10 weeks. Additional time for sessions with the youngster's parents has to be available. The treatment program is costly with regard to the psychologist's time; working with small groups of depressed children makes this a more cost-efficient venture. At the very least, by being able to identify depressed youths and making an appropriate referral, the school psychologist has served the child well.

The Suicidal Child: A Special Case

Any time a child in school reports thoughts about killing him- or herself and the child has thought of specific ways to do it, this is a clear sign of the need to intervene immediately. The objective is to make a successful referral to a mental health clinic. It is extremely important to not minimize the child's suicidal intent. In this case, it may be prudent to err on the conservative side and refer whenever in doubt. Our first step usually is immediately to express our concern to the child about his or her welfare. Additionally, the need to talk to the youngster's parents is explained to the child. It is framed in positive terms as a discussion that will center around what can be done to improve the child's situation. In general, throughout the discussion the clinician emphasizes his or her concern for the child's welfare. Concurrently, the child's parents are called and asked to come immediately in to school to talk about their child. While waiting for the parents to arrive, any apprehensions that the child might have about discussing everyone's concerns about the child hurting him- or herself are addressed, and plans for broaching the topic are discussed and even role-played. Since this period of waiting for the child's parents to arrive is a very stressful time for the child, it is important not to leave the youngster alone even to get a drink or go to the bathroom. The child may act on his or her suicidal intent rather than face his or her parents. On the parents' arrival, a frank discussion ensues in which the child's risk for suicidal behavior is made crystal clear. Ideally, the clinician facilitates the child's self-disclosure about his or her suicidality. Most of the time, the child aids in this endeavor and self-discloses. In those cases where the child will not self-disclose, the therapist is responsible for disclosing the details.

At times, the child does not want his or her parents to be informed. The child may plead with the therapist, get angry, yell, create a scene, or make promises in an attempt to prevent the therapist from informing the child's parents. It is imperative that the therapist not back down. The potential harm to the child and his or her family, the guilt the therapist would feel, as well as possible litigation against the therapist and school district, all portend the immediate contact of the child's parents.

If the child's parents will not arrive for hours and the child is not deemed to be a serious risk, some additional steps are taken. Since this may be a high-stress time for the child that may prompt a suicidal act in a previously nonsuicidal child, steps are taken to ensure the child's safety. Plans are made so that a school official is with the child at all times. If possible, we arrange for an administrator to observe unobtrusively the child passing from class to class. Or the child's teachers are informed and instructed to watch the child pass from one class to the next. If the child goes into the washroom or a lockerroom, a teacher or administrator discreetly follows. If the child's parents can arrive soon enough, the child simply stays in the psychologist's office or in view of the psychologist at all times.

Whenever a child is actively suicidal and warrants the aforementioned action, we recommend to the parents that they immediately take their child to a crisis center with mental health professionals who specialize in working with suicidal clients. A verbal commitment is secured from the parents, and they are warned that their child may try to talk them out of it. Specifically, they are informed that the child may make promises not to ever do it, or the child might say hurtful things. The parents are asked to ignore it for their child's welfare. Commonly the child is either hospitalized for 24 hours for assessment and observation, or the child may be hospitalized for a longer period. Thus, it is important for the parents and child to be aware of this possibility as well as the associated expense.

4

Affective and Cognitive Techniques

OVERVIEW OF A MULTICOMPONENT
TREATMENT PROGRAM

The treatment program that is described in this chapter and the following chapter is based in part on treatment programs that have proven to be effective with depressed adults. Specifically, the treatment programs developed by Beck and colleagues (Beck et al., 1979), Lewinsohn (Lewinsohn & Graf, 1973), and Rehm (Rehm et al., 1987) have been very influential. However, changes have been made to both the content of these treatments and the process of implementing the associated treatment procedures. Changes have been made to reflect the developmental level of the children. In addition, procedures that are more specific to the treatment of children (e.g., Kendall & Braswell, 1985) have been integrated. An attempt has been made to recognize the important role of the family in the development and treatment of depressive disorders. Thus, a family therapy component is an integral part of the treatment program. The process of developing the treatment program has been an extensive one that is based on 5 years of research and clinical experiences with depressed youngsters.

A variety of treatment procedures will be described in the following sections. As noted in Chapter 3, the therapist has to choose the procedures that fit best for each individual child. Typically, a variety of procedures are used with the children and their families. Nonetheless, a number of the procedures seem to form the core of the treatment program and are used across clients.

With the child, a number of cognitive, self-control, and behavioral procedures are used. The cognitive procedures include cognitive restructuring, problem-solving training, cognitive modeling, and strategies for directing attention. The self-control procedures used include self-monitoring, self-consequation, and self-evaluation. The behavioral skills taught to the youngsters include activity scheduling, assertiveness, social skills, and deep muscle relaxation combined with self-administered coping imagery. A number of additional behavioral procedures including education, modeling, role-play, feedback, and social reinforcement are used to teach the aforementioned skills. All of the skills, cognitive, self-control, and behavioral, are taught and used in the therapy sessions and then further mastered and applied *in vivo* through homework assignments. In addition, behavioral contracts and individual or group contingencies are used to help ensure therapeutic compliance.

A key characteristic of cognitive–behavioral procedures is that one of the primary goals of treatment is to teach the child skills so that he or she can control his or her own depressive symptoms. First, the children are given an understanding of the etiology of depression that ties it to the treatment program and helps the youngster understand why he or she is learning the various skills.

AFFECTIVE EDUCATION

Given the fact that the primary disturbance in mood disorders is an affective one, it seems as though it would be important to focus on the youngster's emotionality during treatment. By diagnostic definition, the depressed youngster's affective experience is dominated by either feelings of sadness or a bland, emotionless feeling (anhedonia). In addition, some depressed youngsters (those experiencing dysthymic disorder) report a dominant feeling of anger or irritability. Although these are the predominant emotions, and they are experienced for most of the youngsters' waking hours, there are times when the youngsters feel better. However, these improvements in feelings are often overlooked or forgotten by the children because of an error in information processing. Because of the tendency to see things in dichotomous, all-or-none terms, when depressed children feel some sadness, they allow it to color their entire affective experience. They do not perceive gradations of sadness. Rather, they see themselves as experiencing extreme depression. In addition, because of their tendency to overgeneralize, they give all negative affect the same label. There also are times when a depressed youngster's sadness becomes progressively worse as he or she gets caught up in a downward spiral of dysphoria. It is important for the child to be able to recognize this worsening of sadness, since a change in affect can be used as a cue to introspect or use coping skills. Thus, treatment is directed toward helping the depressed youngster perceive his or her experience of a broader range of affect, to recognize when a change in affect is occurring, and to recognize and correctly label a broad range of emotions.

Recently cognitive therapists have paid greater attention to the role of emotion in the development and maintenance of psychological disorders, and they have begun developing therapeutic strategies for directly intervening at the level of the maladaptive affect. Affective education programs have been the primary vehicle for promoting this change. During affective education, the youngster is taught the labels for a wide variety of emotions, both pleasant and unpleasant. The youngster also is taught that each emotion is experienced along a continuum of the intensity of experience. Finally, they are taught to recognize and label their own affective experiences. As a consequence of this affective education, the child also learns to identify the emotional state of others in his or her environment.

A number of activities are used as an enjoyable vehicle for teaching the children about emotions. The activities begin educating the children at a basic level and then build on this knowledge in a logical fashion. The youngsters are taught increasingly complex skills and to make increasingly finer distinctions between emotions. In addition to providing the youngsters with a better understanding of their emotions, the activities also serve as the vehicle for teaching the youngsters the relationship among thoughts, feelings, and behaviors. Thus, the rationale for treatment is established during these early sessions. The affective education activities serve another purpose. They are used during the early sessions to help the youngster(s) get used to disclosing personal information. They help establish a sense of trust. When a group format is used for delivering the treatment program, these activities are used to establish group cohesion. Experience indicates that this sense of group cohesion is a necessity for the success of the group treatment format.

The list of activities that comprise the affective education program are listed in Table 4.1. The first activity, emotional vocabulary, is designed at the most basic level to teach the child a vocabulary for emotions. At another level, the youngsters learn that there are a wide variety of emotions. The first step in the procedure is to develop a list of names of emotions that are appropriate for the intellectual level of the client. A partial list of names of emotions can be found in

TABLE 4.1. Sequence of Activities Used in the Affective Education Program

1. *Emotion vocabulary*

   Players take turns choosing emotion cards and reading aloud the name of the emotion on the card. Then the player describes how the emotion feels and what was happening the last time he or she experienced the emotion.

2. *Emotion vocabulary II*

   Players read the name of the emotion aloud and then describe what a person who is experiencing the emotion might be thinking and how he or she might be behaving.

3. *Emotion charades*

   After silently reading the card, each player thinks about how a person who feels that way looks and how he or she might behave. Then the player acts out the emotion without saying anything or making any noises. The other players guess the name of the emotion being acted out.

4. *Emotion statues*

   Players take turns playing the sculptor, the statue, and the audience. The sculptor picks a card and then shapes the statue's facial expression, arms, hands, feet, and legs to express the emotion. The audience guesses the name of the emotion.

5. *Emotion expression*

   Players take turns drawing cards from the deck and reading them silently. The actor expresses the emotion through making noises while the other players try to guess the name of the emotion.

Table 4.2. This list should be expanded for use with older children and adolescents, and the list may be reduced for younger children (below 10 years). The next step is to write the name of each emotion on a 3-by-5 card. Given the heavy use of the cards, it is prudent to have them laminated. The deck of cards is then used to play the game. The therapist and youngster(s) take turns blindly picking

TABLE 4.2. List of Emotions That Can Be Used in the Affective Education Activities

Happy	Hurt	Upset
Mad	Furious	Guilty
Sad	Jealous	Left out
Scared	Nervous	Put down
Surprised	Ashamed	Discouraged
Lonely	Excited	Relieved
Bored	Frustrated	Confused
Proud		

cards from the deck. After choosing a card, the player reads the name of the emotion out loud. Then, the player describes how the emotion feels and what was happening the last time he or she experienced that emotion. After going through the deck, the deck is shuffled, and the game continues until the youngster(s) have mastered the emotion vocabulary. Mastery is attained when the child can accurately describe each emotion in the deck.

During Emotional Vocabulary II, the relationship among thought, emotion, and behavior is established. This is accomplished by once again using the cards with the emotions written on them. The players take turns blindly picking cards from the deck. This time the players read the name of the emotion aloud and then describe what a person who is experiencing the emotion might be thinking and how he or she might be behaving. More often than not, the therapist has to spend a good deal of time coaching the youngster(s) through this process. Children usually do not associate specific thoughts with specific emotions. Rather, they tend to see emotions as simply arising out of thin air. By starting to link thought and emotion, the children get an idea of the types of thoughts they might be having that lead to their unpleasant emotions. It also helps them learn that the source of their sadness is their thoughts and that these thoughts can be controlled. This sense of control can lead to an improvement in symptomatology.

The deck of cards used in the previous two activities is also used in emotion charades, which is the third game. This time, the players take turns drawing cards from the deck, but they read them to themselves rather than aloud. After reading the card, the player thinks about how a person who feels that way looks and how he or she might behave. Then the player acts out the emotion without saying anything or making any noises. The other players take turns guessing the name of the emotion being acted out. If the emotion is not correctly identified, then the actor is encouraged to try new ways of expressing the emotions, and the game continues until the emotion is correctly identified. When the emotion is correctly identified, the player states what the actor did that led him or her to identify the emotion correctly. In addition, the player states what was happening or might have been happening the last time he or she felt that way *and* what he or she was thinking at that time.

Some emotions are difficult to act out and identify through their overt expression. Thus, it is useful to allow and encourage the players to help each other in such situations. This is important, since one of the goals of the activity is for the child to enjoy him- or herself as well as to learn about emotions. As a result of this activity, the child learns how to identify the emotional state of significant others in his or her environment. This skill is used by the child later in therapy when the child is trying to change his or her environment.

The fourth activity in the series is emotion statues. This activity works best with a group of children. It is inappropriate for use with an individual child. Once again, the deck of emotion cards is used. This time the players take turns playing the sculptor, the statue, and the audience. The sculptor or sculptors (since this can be a difficult task, we commonly use multiple sculptors to ensure success) shape the person playing the statue into an expression of the emotion. They shape the statue's facial expression and the placement of his or her arms, hands, feet, and legs. The other group members guess the name of the emotion. Once correctly identified, the player states what a person experiencing that emotion is likely to be thinking and what might have been happening. If the youngster has experienced that emotion before, he or she is asked to describe what he or she was thinking and what was happening. This activity seems to be the favorite one, since many youngsters ask to play it again later in treatment.

The final activity is emotion expression. During this activity, the players take turns drawing cards from the deck and reading them silently. Then, the actor expresses the emotion auditorily. He or she tries to express the emotion through his or her voice. No words are used. The children try to express the emotion in their voices through the noises they make. The other players try to guess the emotion. Once the emotion has been accurately identified, the person who identified the emotion states what the cues were in the actor's voice that helped him or her identify it. Then the child describes the last time he or she felt that way, what thoughts he or she had, and what was happening. Once again, this activity helps the youngster learn more about his or her emotions, the cognition–affect link, and how to identify the emotional state of significant others in his or her life.

While the children are playing the games, the therapist attempts to help the children recognize the continuum of severity of emotions. This can be accomplished by pointing out how the different names of emotions can note different levels of severity. In addition, the therapist asks questions about the child's reported experience of an emotion. These questions help the child see that there are different levels of severity and that he or she experiences the emotions differently at different times. For example, the therapist might ask the child to compare how he or she was feeling during this incident relative to another incident that was reported during an earlier game.

COGNITIVE TECHNIQUES

The cognitive techniques are an integral part of the treatment program. They are used by the therapist throughout the course of treatment, and a number of sessions have to be devoted solely to cognitive techniques. There are a few general rules that are followed when teaching them to the children. First, the therapist and child client move from collecting and restructuring automatic thoughts that seem to occur in isolation or randomly to watching for and identifying themes in these thoughts that are reflective of maladaptive cognitive structures or core cognitive structures. Second, the therapist begins using the techniques in a tentative, probing fashion as he or she tests the youngster's readiness for change. As treatment progresses and the client is ready for greater attention to his or her thinking, the client and therapist vigorously attack maladaptive cognitions. Third, in the beginning of treatment, the therapist is primarily responsible for identifying and restructuring the client's maladaptive cognitions. Over the course of treatment, the client is taught to identify his or her own maladaptive thoughts and beliefs and to restructure them. Fourth, the goal of treatment is to produce deep, seemingly philosophical change. The youngster learns a new, more adaptive way of constructing his or her perceptions of the world. Fifth, the most powerful way to produce cognitive change is to strategically alter behavior in a fashion that directly restructures the premises underlying the cognitions. Through behavioral assignments, maladaptive cognitions and cognitive structures are diminished, and new more adaptive ones are constructed. Finally, over the course of treatment, core cognitive structures are revealed and become the focus of change.

Cognitive Restructuring

Cognitive restructuring procedures are designed to modify the client's thinking and the premises, assumptions, and attitudes underlying the client's thoughts (Meichenbaum, 1977). They are designed to change the way the client derives meaning from the world. Mahoney and Arnkoff (1978) noted that three primary cognitive restructuring approaches have emerged, including cognitive therapy (e.g., Beck et al., 1979), rational emotive therapy (e.g., Ellis, 1962), and self-instructional training (Meichenbaum, 1977).

Of these three approaches to cognitive restructuring, only the self-instructional training procedure has received widespread use and empirical evaluation with children. This procedure can be used when treating depressed youths, but it is not the preferred or most commonly used method. Self-instructional training traditionally has been used with children who exhibit a deficit in their thinking. In other words, the child's problems appear to result from the fact that the youngster fails to employ cognitive strategies or to think certain thoughts that guide his or her behavior. This procedure has primarily been used with children who exhibit externalizing disorders. It is assumed that these youngsters fail to control their behavior because they lack the mediational strategies to do so (e.g., Kendall, 1985).

As noted in Chapter 2, there has been some research (Butler et al., 1980) that has been directed toward evaluating the effectiveness of a rational emotive approach to cognitive restructuring as a treatment for depression in children. Results of this investigation indicated that the procedure was moderately effective. We do not use Ellis's disputational cognitive restructuring procedures with children because they have a tendency to perceive them as scolding. One youngster said to a practicum student, "You sound just like my parents — always griping at me." Children, especially depressed children, personalize the disputing rather than perceive it as a procedure for gauging the rationality of their thinking. Children and adolescents have a harder time than adults distancing themselves from their thoughts.

Beck's approach to cognitive restructuring has been used most widely in our treatment program. This approach involves four techniques, all of which are designed to help the client change the cognitive structures that underlie his or her maladaptive thoughts. The four techniques are: (1) "What's the evidence?" (2) "What are alternative ways of looking at it?" (3) "What if?" and (4) behavioral assignments that are designed to test directly the premises underlying the cognitive structures. These four procedures and self-instructional training will be described in some detail in the sections that follow. In addition, a problem-solving procedure and a cognitive modeling procedure will be described. However, before this discussion, methods for identifying depressogenic cognitions and cognitive structures will be described.

Identification of Maladaptive Cognitions

The first step of cognitive restructuring is the identification of maladaptive thoughts and the cognitive structures that underlie them. With children, this can be a difficult task. Nonetheless, it is the first step, and success at this stage is a prerequisite to the successful implementation of the treatment procedures.

A number of procedures are used to identify and collect depresso-genic thoughts from children. The first method relies heavily on the therapist's skills. The therapist listens to the content of the child's statements during therapy sessions. The therapist listens for state-ments, especially ones of a self-evaluative nature, that are unrealisti-cally negative and are associated with negative affect. Usually these statements are extreme and include such words as "all," "everyone," "no one," "everything," "anything," "never," "always," "must," and "have to." Sometimes the child says so many unrealistically negative thoughts that the therapist has to collect (write them down) and save them for future reference. It is assumed that the child's statements are a direct reflection of his or her thoughts. For example, it is assumed that a child who says "I'm no good at anything," "Everyone hates me," "I'm going to fail," truly believes these things, and it is assumed that the statements are direct reflections of his or her thoughts. If these statements are not true, then they may reflect a distorted style of thinking that becomes the target of cognitive re-structuring.

Another procedure involves simply asking the child what he or she was thinking about at certain times. More specifically, when the child relays a story about an experience, the therapist inquires about what the child was thinking at that time. For example, a child relays the story to the therapist about her parents telling her that she needed to choose which one she wants to live with, since they are breaking up. The therapist may ask the child to explain what was happening and what she was thinking about during this time. What did the child think led to the split, and what role did she think she had played in it? What did she think was going to happen next? What process was she following to make her decision? Would things work out for her? Will she always feel this bad? What can she do to help herself feel better? What things has she done in the past to make herself feel better? What does it mean to her to have this happen? Additional questions and probing would be used as necessary to gain a thorough understanding of the child's perceptions about what was happening, how it would impact her life, and what it meant about her. Since children often respond to such direct questions with "I don't know" or minimal responses, a good deal of probing is com-monly necessary. In addition, the questions may need to be even more closed-ended. The therapist may have to project what the youngster may have been thinking and then ask the child to verify the accuracy of these thoughts. For example: "You were thinking that they only cared about themselves and not you?"

A more structured procedure that we have followed is to ask the child to indicate, from among a list of thoughts, the ones that he or she has. A copy of such a list is far from complete. Any thoughts can be included. Oftentimes it is useful to consider everything you know about the child and then construct a list of thoughts that the child might have in areas that are of concern to him or her. After the child completes the list, the therapist reviews the list and looks for patterns in the thoughts. For example, a theme of only being of value when others like you may become evident. These patterns of thoughts become the target of change. If the therapist is uncertain about the validity of the results, then they are used to form hypotheses that are tested by using other assessment procedures.

One of the most commonly used techniques is to ask the child to self-monitor his or her thoughts and then write them down. Commonly, the child is asked to use a change in mood, the occurrence of a specific event, or the occurrence of a specific type of thought as a cue to record what he or she was thinking. The degree of structure used to help the child complete the self-monitoring varies. The author has used a highly structured approach. A form has been constructed that facilitates the process. A copy of this form can be found in Appendix D. The child is asked to use a change in mood as a cue to record what was happening and what he or she was thinking. As can be seen in Appendix D, the form has the emotional stimulus typed on it along with two questions that serve as prompts: "What was happening?" and "What I am thinking?" After each cue question is space for the child to record his or her responses to the questions. The child is given at least one of these forms to complete for each day that will pass between sessions. The forms are compiled in a three-ring binder that the child carries around with him- or herself. The completed forms are removed and kept by the therapist. The therapist and child review them at the beginning of each session.

These forms can be altered to suit each youngster's needs. The specific cue question for the child may be recorded along with any additional necessary prompts. The younger the child, the more structured the form, in other words, the more information that is included on the form. Since these forms are commonly referred to in later sessions, and since children commonly mix up or lose things, it is recommended that the forms have a place to record the date and the day of the week that they were completed. With some youngsters, those who are young or more forgetful, the therapist will ask one of the youngster's parents to help by filling in this information. At other times, the therapist might fill in this information prior to giving the child the forms. With children who are resistant to directly revealing what they are thinking, or for children who simply do not talk a lot, other procedures may have to be used to elicit their thoughts. Projective techniques are especially helpful with such youngsters. Projective techniques including a thorough inquiry stage are used like a semi-structured interview to obtain information about the child's thinking (Prout & Ferber, 1988). The content of the stimulus should be chosen so that it elicits the information that is of concern. For example, if the therapist is concerned about the child's thoughts in social situations, a picture from a book, magazine, or cartoon that portrays a social situation may be chosen, or a card from the Roberts Apperception Test might be used. The child is shown the picture, which is followed by a period of inquiry including questions about what the child in the picture is thinking and feeling. Further probing can be used to gain a better understanding of what the youngster believes is happening, what happened before, what will happen next, and anything else that will help to clarify the child's thoughts in such situations.

Similarly, other projective techniques can be used to gain an understanding of the child's way of constructing his or her world. Incomplete sentences, play, and drawings can be used. A minimum of interpretation is used when one is trying to understand the child's responses to the stimulus materials. The child's responses are directly interpreted as being a reflection of his or her own thinking. This low level of interpretation is most appropriate and easily applied when the youngster begins to refer to the cases in a way that suggests that he or she is personalizing the response. For example, the child might start saying "I," "me," or "mine" while describing the scene. In other cases where the child refers to the main character as the "boy" or "girl" in the picture, it is inferred that the child is really placing his or her own construction on the stimulus. Thus, the child's responses are still directly interpreted as a reflection of his or her thinking. There is no attempt in either case to interpret symbols as representative of underlying processes.

Identification of Cognitive Structures and Core

The key to successful cognitive therapy is the identification and modification of the client's cognitive structures and core cognitive structures. Meaningful and long-lasting change will occur only if change is achieved at this level. Changing the youngster's cognitive structures, especially his or her core cognitive structures, changes the way the child derives meaning from the world. It changes what the child attends to and how he or she interprets or structures incoming information. It is this depth of change that serves as the goal of treatment.

Safran, Vallis, Segal, and Shaw (1986) have identified two types of cognitive assessment that they refer to as horizontal and vertical assessment. Horizontal assessment is a more surface level assessment process. It is a process that involves eliciting and exploring the range of automatic thoughts that surround a given situation or emotional reaction. The therapist and child-client work together to identify the thoughts the child had before, during, or after a particular event or emotional reaction. Any of the procedures noted in the previous section can be used to elicit the thoughts. This assessment process reveals for the client and therapist the range of maladaptive thoughts that the child is experiencing. In horizontal assessment, the therapist intervenes after identifying a maladaptive thought.

Vertical assessment, in contrast, is a deeper level of assessment than horizontal assessment. Like horizontal assessment, it is a hypothesis generation and testing process. However, it involves some inference on the part of the therapist. Vertical assessment begins in a similar manner to horizontal assessment. However, during the process of assessing the range of cognitions, the therapist forms hypotheses about what might be underlying the thoughts. During vertical assessment, the therapist does not intervene after identifying maladaptive thoughts. Rather, the therapist continues to explore the client's cognitions and waits to intervene until after a tacit rule that would explain the cognitions that have been identified. Then, the core cognitive structure that is assumed to underlie the rule becomes the target of the cognitive restructuring.

As Safran and colleagues (1986) note, this hypothesis generation and assessment process is guided by a number of rules. First, the therapist develops hypotheses about the thematic nature of the cognitions. For example, the child might express a theme of being unworthy or undeserving of help. The therapist might try to identify redundancies in the content of the child-client's thoughts and images. For example, a child might report over and over a lack of ties with other children. In addition, the therapist identifies consistencies in the child's behaviors (e.g., isolating oneself from social contact) and emotional reactions. Finally, consistencies in the situations that are associated with maladaptive thoughts and emotions are identified (e.g., interpersonal situations).

Cognitions that are associated with, or have implications for, the self tend to be more central or core to the individual. It is assumed (Safran et al., 1986) that cognitive structures about the self are more primal in the developmental process. Thus, they are referred to as core cognitive structures. They account for a broader range of behaviors and emotional responses. Particularly important are cognitions that involve an evaluation of the self. In addition, thoughts that are an evaluation of the impact of an event on the perception of the self are more central. The therapist also tries to ascertain the meaning of a predicted (client predicted) event for the client's self-perception, for example, "What would it mean about you if she didn't want to meet you at the dance?"

Another rule to follow for identifying core cognitions is to watch for changes in the client's affect. Once the change in affect occurs, the therapist notes the content of the cognitions that were being discussed. If the discussion was not centering around specific thoughts at the time of the change, then the therapist redirects the focus of therapy to the thoughts and images the client was having just before he or she became emotional. The child is asked to take a few moments to try to reflect back to those thoughts and to reconstruct them. The therapist may have to help the child reconstruct the discussion that led up to the emotional reaction.

Implementation Issues

As noted in Chapter 3, an empathic understanding of the client is essential for the successful implementation of cognitive restructuring techniques. This understanding guides the therapist's efforts to restructure the client's thinking and the organizing principles (cognitive structures) underlying these thoughts. It is unwise to begin implementing cognitive restructuring procedures prior to the point in time when the therapist has gained such an understanding of the child-client. The exception to this rule is the child who is in crisis (e.g., suicidal). In such cases, the therapist has to be more active and has to promote some immediate relief.

Early in the treatment of a depressed youth, the child usually is unready for cognitive restructuring. Typically, the child seems unwilling to entertain the possibility that his or her thoughts are erroneous. Instead, the youngster holds on to his or her thoughts. Research indicates that people do not process information that is inconsistent with their cognitive structures (for a review see Turk & Salovey, 1985). At other times the youngster may be too busy telling his or her story to hear and consider what the therapist has to say. The child may be obsessed with depressogenic thoughts (thoughts that are associated with depressive symptoms). At this time, it is unwise to begin cognitive restructuring because it would just add to the youngster's already cluttered stream of consciousness. Having the child think about his or her depressive thoughts would just feed the child's depression. It is better to wait until the child has acquired some coping skills for controlling his or her depressive symptoms prior to using cognitive restructuring procedures.

Another consideration when deciding when to begin cognitive restructuring is where you are in the assessment process. Have you listened and questioned enough to have completed a vertical assessment? Have you identified core cognitive structures, and have you verified the validity of these core cognitive structures for the child? If the therapist restructures more surface-level cognitions and cognitive structures, the impact will be short-lived. The therapist can scurry around changing these surface-level thoughts producing short-term symptom improvement, whereas changing core cognitive structures and cognitive structures leads to long-lasting change. Thus, it is important not to intervene too early before the core cognitive structures have been identified. Intervening too early also might lead to some short-term changes that might hinder the assessment process.

How does a therapist know that it is an appropriate time to begin cognitive restructuring? Similarly to other procedures, the therapist watches for communications from the client that he or she is ready. The child-client is ready when he or she demonstrates some control over his or her symptoms. At this time, the child can better cope with the increased attention to maladaptive cognitions. In addition, the child may be able to gain some objectivity at this time that helps the youngster see the fallacy of his or her thinking.

A procedure that can be used to gauge readiness is to do some testing of the child's readiness for cognitive restructuring. This can be accomplished by identifying a maladaptive cognition and challenging its premise. If the child demonstrates the ability to listen and process what is being discussed, the child may be ready for cognitive restructuring to begin. When the child no longer talks over the therapist, he or she may be ready. Another good indication is when the child responds by contemplating what the therapist has said rather than immediately discounting or denying it. At first, this often is the best that can be expected. Over time, the therapist keeps chipping away at the child's maladaptive cognitive structures. Another very good sign is when the youngster is willing to try on the therapist's hypothesis to determine whether it makes sense for him- or herself. Another good sign is when the child reports spontaneously coming up with alternative thoughts between sessions. Finally, when the child begins to question him- or herself in a similar fashion to the therapist, the child is starting to change. The child may also show some acceptance of the therapist's proposed alternative conceptualizations.

Some cautions also are in order. If the child appears to accept the therapist's reframe or more adaptive way of deriving meaning from events without question, then the youngster may be just agreeing with the therapist without really changing his or her thinking. The therapist should beware of such quick agreements. These children may be agreeing with the therapist at the time, but they quickly forget or go back to their old style of thinking on leaving the therapist's office. Cognitive change takes time and work on the client's part. It is less likely to occur when a child passively sits, listens, and thoughtlessly agrees with the therapist.

It is important to remember that the goal of cognitive restructuring is to produce deep, philosophical change. Such change only occurs when core cognitive structures have been changed. Thus, these more core structures should command the therapist's attention.

Cognitive–behavioral therapies tend to be short-term therapies. This has implications for cognitive restructuring. Since it would take a great deal of time, and since the therapist wants the child to become independent as soon as possible, it is important for the child to learn how to identify his or her own maladaptive thinking and the underlying premises. Once identified, the child asks him- or herself the same questions that the therapist asks. It is at this point, when the child is acting as his or her own cognitive therapist, that therapy is a success. It is this latter stage of cognitive restructuring that therapists commonly fail to build into their treatment goals. Consequently, they fail to produce long-term change.

Cognitive Restructuring Procedures

While one is trying to implement the cognitive restructuring procedures, it is important to keep two principles foremost in mind. First one should remember that the primary target of change is the youngster's core cognitive structures. The second principle is the long-term goal of teaching the child to apply these procedures independently to his or her own maladaptive cognitions.

"What's the evidence?" Developed by Beck and Emery (1985), "What's the evidence?" may be one of the most useful and easily applied cognitive restructuring procedures. The nature of the procedure is captured in its title. It involves asking the child to work with the therapist to identify the evidence that supports or refutes his or

her automatic thoughts and the cognitive structures underlying them. The child and therapist collaboratively identify maladaptive thoughts and the cognitive structures or core cognitive structures that are associated with depressive symptoms. This process may involve any of the assessment procedures mentioned earlier. Frequently, they appear in the things the child discusses during the interview. As noted earlier, the objective of the assessment is to continue to explore the depth and breadth of these thoughts. Once the core cognitions have been identified, the therapist asks the child to identify the evidence that supports (it is assumed that a minimum of supportive evidence will be found) *and* refutes the core cognitive structure. Prior to using "What's the evidence?" the therapist must know the child well enough to be sure that the targeted cognitive structure does not reflect reality. If it does reflect reality, then this procedure should not be used. Problem solving and "What if" should be used instead. Mistakenly asking the child to provide evidence that supports a maladaptive cognitive structure is counterproductive.

When the therapist was working with a depressed boy and his formerly depressed single-parent mother, a maladaptive cognitive structure became apparent over the course of a couple of sessions, and "What's the evidence?" was used to restructure the boy's thinking. Before describing the implementation of the procedure, some additional background information is necessary. Over the course of a couple of years, the boy's mother had experienced a number of major stressful events. First, this boy's parents had divorced after the mother decided she had had all she could tolerate of the father's alcohol abuse. Subsequently, she entered another relationship that eventually failed for a relatively long period of time. The boy's recollections of this time were of his mother crying, being withdrawn, and spending a great deal of time just lying on the sofa not feeling up to doing anything. They experienced a good deal of financial hardship, and the boy's emotional needs were not being fulfilled. Travis increasingly assumed responsibility for taking care of his mother. His cognitive structure of his mother was that of a fragile individual who needed to be cared for or else she would fall apart. At the time that I began working with Travis and his mother, his mother had overcome her depression and was quite vigorous. Nonetheless, Travis continued to perceive his mother as weak and helpless.

The therapist proceeded to engage Travis in "What's the evidence?" The therapist first determined the validity of the hypothesis that his mother was weak. This was accomplished simply by restating Travis' remarks that led to the hypothesis and then verbalizing the premise underlying these remarks. Travis agreed with the therapist that he thought of his mother as weak and needing of his care. Next, the therapist asked Travis to describe how his mother would have to behave in order to be considered weak. After Travis stated the necessary evidence to support this contention (e.g., cries a lot, gets hurt frequently, can't do things), the therapist then guided him through the process of questioning the validity of each premise. During this process, the therapist kept Travis focused on his mother's behavior over the past 6 months: "Has your mom cried lately? Does she stay home from work? Has house-cleaning been neglected? Have you had to make your own meals?" and so forth. As each question was tested, the therapist and Travis evaluated the evidence, and it consistently contradicted the weakness premise. Next, the evidence for the contrary premise (mom is in fact a strong woman) was evaluated. This time the therapist led Travis through a series of questions that provided evidence that supported the fact that she was strong (e.g., she smiled a lot, wasn't seen crying, went to work regularly, made him meals).

During this process, the therapist took notes, and after it was over, Travis and the therapist reviewed all of the evidence and the therapist asked the question, "Does your mom seem to be strong or weak?" The reply was "strong." This was followed by some educating of Travis about his mother's, and for that matter anyone's, reaction to the loss of a spouse. Travis' mother was actively involved in this process as she provided evidence for the strength argument. Finally, the therapist said that it was necessary to test further the new hypothesis that his mother was strong. He was asked to collect evidence over the next week that would support the contention that his mom was strong. Whenever he came across an incident that provided evidence for his mom being strong, he was asked to record it on a sheet of paper and to bring the list to the next meeting.

The previous example represents a preliminary attempt to use "What's the evidence?" It was effective at producing immediate symptom relief. However, for long-term change, it is necessary to teach the child to ask him- or herself to identify depressogenic thoughts and then ask "What's the evidence for the thoughts?" This is accomplished over time as the therapist models the procedure. For example, a seventh-grade boy named Matt was referred for social skills training directed toward helping him to fit in better with his peers and to stop getting into fights. One of Matt's core beliefs was that the other kids were out to humiliate him. He believed that they (his peers) were plotting to humiliate him publicly. Matt considered public humiliation to be the worst possible thing that could happen. Fighting, even if it meant getting beaten up or suspended from school, was a lesser consequence than public humiliation. The choice of the maladaptive cognitive structure to work on was difficult because Matt had so many that they pervaded most of the things that he said. Nevertheless, the most disconcerting one became the target.

Each session, Matt came in to the office complaining about the way he was being treated by his peers. At first the therapist spent most of his time listening to Matt, eliciting historical information about his friendships, and in general trying to gain a better understanding of Matt and the way he thinks about himself and the world in general. It took a number of sessions before Matt could gain enough distance from his thoughts to be able to benefit from cognitive restructuring. The therapist gently queried about the evidence supporting the notion that the other kids, "*all*" of the other kids, were out to humiliate him. As it became evident that Matt was capable of doubting that *everyone* was trying to humiliate him, the therapist became more confrontational in his questioning and pointed out that Matt was thinking in "all or nothing" terms. In addition, the therapist helped Matt to see how his thinking about his peers and social situations was impacting his social life and overall sense of contentment. Finally, Matt was taught to ask himself "What's the evidence?" every time he began to feel as though the other kids disliked him or that they were out to humiliate him. If Matt had just been taught to ask himself the question, he would have continued to believe that they were out to humiliate him. He also had to be taught what would constitute evidence that would support and contradict his contention.

To help children understand this process of evaluating the evidence, an analogy to being a detective is used with the child. The youngster is given a cartoon (see Figure 4.1) that has two children dressed in traditional detective clothing. This is followed by a discussion about what a detective does and how he or she collects evidence. The child is taught to be a thought detective who goes around collecting the evidence for his or her maladaptive thoughts.

Alternative Interpretations. The depressed child tends to have a narrow and negativistic way of processing information. Alternative interpretations is a procedure that is designed to broaden the focus of the client's thinking (Beck & Emery, 1985). When using alternative interpretations, the therapist and child work together to develop alternative interpretations/constructions of the upsetting event. It is assumed that if the negativistic interpretation is replaced with a more positive and adaptive one, the child will feel better. Once again it is important to emphasize that the therapist and child are not

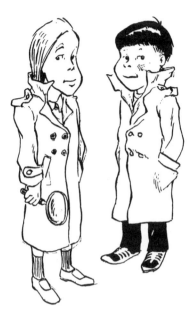

FIGURE 4.1. Detective cartoon.

trying to develop a fantasy world of positive perceptions that masks reality; in contrast, it is believed that the child is misconstruing reality and that the collaborative effort is designed to help the child develop new, more realistic interpretations of what is happening in his or her life. For example, early teens commonly complain that "Mary hates me. I was walking down the hall today, and she didn't even say 'Hi' to me. She acted like I didn't even exist." This failure to return the salutation could have resulted from a number of factors, thus leading to a number of possible constructions being placed on the incident. The youngster has made the following interpretation — Mary did not say "Hi." Therefore, she hates me. There are a variety of other possible reasons why Mary did not say "Hi." Mary might not have heard you say "Hi." Maybe Mary was talking with someone else. Perhaps she was thinking about something that had just happened. Maybe she was angry with you, but that does not mean that she hates you. Could Mary have been trying to remember the homework assignment she had been given? Could she have been spacing out? Any one of these interpretations is a possibility.

Middle-school children commonly express humor through cutting one-liners — a practice that is consistent with current modes of communication among characters on television. The cut-downs typically are not meant to be taken personally. Rather, they are thoughtless statements that are designed for everyone's humor and to elicit attention for the speaker. Most teens blow off such cutting comments as playful interchange. Depressed children, in contrast, often take such comments personally. They tend to believe the cutting comment or that the speaker does not like them and made the comment to be mean. When dealing with depressed children who take such comments personally, alternative interpretations can be used. For example, Matt would commonly complain about the other kids hating him, and his proof was the one-liners that some of his peers were saying. The task became one of opening Matt's eyes to alternative ways of interpreting the one-liners. The therapist asked Matt whether it was possible that the person who made the cutting comment was doing it for some reason other than because he hated you. Could he have said it just to be funny? Could he have said it just because that is what he says to everyone? Do kids your age joke around by saying such things? Have you and your friends exchanged cuts in good humor before?

"What If?" Sometimes the child is in a difficult and disappointing situation. In such situations, the depressed child often exaggerates the significance of the situation, or the child may predict unrealistically dire outcomes. When this occurs, "What if" (Beck et al., 1979) can be a useful procedure. The objective of the procedure is to help the child gain a more realistic perspective on the meaning of the situation for the child. In addition, when the child is predicting an unrealistically negative outcome, "What if" can be used to help the child realize that the actual outcome is likely to be less dire.

When using this procedure, it is important to note that the procedure has to be implemented in a sincere and nonsarcastic fashion. It is important for a solid client–therapist relationship to be in existence when this procedure is being used. This helps ensure that the child does not perceive the therapists' comments as being sarcastic or as being representative of the fact that the therapist "does not understand" the child and/or his situation.

When using "What if," the therapist agrees with the objective facts about the situation and about the distressing nature of the situation. However, the therapist listens for examples of the child's thinking that indicate that the child is exaggerating the significance of the situation for him- or herself. For example, an eighth-grade boy was extremely distraught because his girlfriend was moving to a different city. As a result of the move, the youngster would only be able to see her on special occasions. The boy kept saying that he probably would never see her again, that she would move, find another boy-friend and not want anything to do with him. As a result of not being able to see her, his time would be spent isolated and lonely — no one would be there who would care about him. Thus, underlying his sadness was the belief that he had to be with her or he was destined to a life of loneliness. This was then countered by using "What's the evidence?"

As the children master the three primary cognitive restructuring procedures (What's the evidence?, alternative interpretations, and What if?), a shift is made to a more comprehensive self-monitoring form. A copy of this form can be found in Appendix E. A comparison of the simpler form found in Appendix D with this form, reveals that there are additional prompts that facilitate both self-monitoring (What was happening? What was I doing? What were my thoughts?) and cognitive restructuring (the evidence, alternatives, my choice). The form was designed to be a guide to the independent use of the cognitive restructuring procedures. As the child confronts a problematic emotion, he or she notes what was happening and what he or she was doing, thus helping the child learn the role that he or she is playing in the occurrence of various problematic situations. Then the child introspects and writes down his or her thoughts. Next the youngster writes down the evidence that supports or contradicts the thoughts. Subsequently, possible alternative interpretations of the situation are generated. Finally, the child chooses an alternative interpretation or a new thought based on the evidence. Once again, the therapist reviews these forms at the beginning of each session.

Behavioral Assignments. Perhaps the most powerful way to change an individual's thinking is to change his or her related behavior (Meichenbaum, 1977). Changing thinking through changing related behavior provides the child with immediate, direct, and concrete evidence that addresses the validity of the youngster's cognitive structures. Although this procedure provides the child with immediate, direct, and concrete feedback, it still is possible for the child to misconstrue the results of the behavioral assignment. Thus, it is important for the therapist to process the results with the child. During this processing, the therapist reviews the results of the assignment and points out schema-inconsistent information.

During work with a depressed eighth-grade female, the subject complained about numerous aspects of her appearance. She saw herself as fat, ugly, and as having ugly hair. To test the belief that she was fat, the following procedure was used. First, the therapist helped the child to define overt evidence that someone is overweight. For example, the person would have cellulite wrinkles in her hips. The person would have loose, hanging flesh. The person would have large quantities of flesh that bulged out from the skeleton. Examples for each criterion were solicited from the child to tighten up the evidence.

Following the therapy session, the girl attended P.E. This required undressing, locking one's clothes in a locker, and showering. The girl was asked if there was anyone in her P.E. class who was overweight. She named the individual, and the therapist determined which of the aforementioned criteria of being overweight she met. Once these criteria were firmly established, the therapist worked out a plan for testing the belief that she was fat. During her P.E. class she would choose a locker next to the overweight girl. When the two of them changed, she would compare her figure on each of the criteria to that of the other girl. After the P.E. class, she reported back to the school psychologist's office and processed the results of the assignment. She concluded that she was not "fat."

A sixth-grade depressed boy had fallen far behind in his schoolwork. He experienced a lot of fatigue and believed that he was too "stupid" to successfully complete the work and that it was not worth the effort to try, since he was going to fail anyway. One of the goals of treatment, at least from the parents', school's, and to some extent the child's perspective, was to increase the quality and quantity of completed homework. To this end, the therapist created an assignment that would test Jamie's belief that he could not complete his schoolwork. Jamie was given a pass to go and get his natural science book. This was a class that Jamie enjoyed and had performed quite well in before his depressive episode. On his return, the therapist and Jamie reviewed his belief that he was incapable of completing his homework. Subsequently, the therapist asked him to pull out his homework sheet. Then Jamie was asked to read the first question aloud. The therapist encouraged Jamie to try to find the answer. With some encouragement and prompts he was successful. This procedure continued with the therapist slowly fading his involvement. With each success, Jamie's mood appeared to improve. Jamie was encouraged to try to complete some of his homework on his own that evening and to call the therapist during the time that he worked on his homework. The goal for Jamie was simply to attempt to do a few problems in a class of choice.

A couple of days later Jamie and the school psychologist met and once again worked on Jamie's homework. Since Jamie was successful at completing his homework with the therapist's help, he became aware that he was capable of completing his schoolwork but that he was quite far behind and that it required a good deal of effort on his part to catch up. Tutorials were scheduled with his teachers as part of the plan to help him get caught up. Jamie and the therapist continued to complete some homework during a portion of each session. The remainder of the session was spent working on other more emotionally laden issues.

Cognitive Modeling. One of the more subtle and effective treatment procedures that can be used to treat depressed youths is cognitive modeling. This procedure is used throughout treatment and involves the therapist verbalizing his or her thoughts. The therapist verbalizes his or her thoughts about various problematic or emotional situations. In addition, the therapist models alternative, more adaptive thoughts that the child could use in problematic situations or situations that are associated with depression. Although this would appear to be a simple procedure, it actually requires a fair amount of skill. The therapist has to develop a natural style of quickly verbalizing coping thoughts. These thoughts have to be developmentally appropriate and realistic for the child. For example, while two student therapists were working with a small group of depressed elementary-aged children, one of the student therapists locked his keys in the car, causing them to be late to group that day. The therapists used this situation to model their own problem-solving thoughts as well as thoughts that the children could have had to cope with the disappointment of not knowing whether they were going to meet that day.

When the therapists arrived, they gathered the children and explained what had happened that had led to their late arrival. Eric explained that he had accidentally locked his keys in the car. He noted that he was frustrated because it seemed like such a stupid act. His frustration was heightened by the fact that he could look in the window and see his keys just a couple of feet away. He noted that he also felt concerned because he thought that the kids in the group would be disappointed and upset about missing the meeting. Then,

> I thought, wait a minute, there is no need to panic. The problem is that I want to get to Northwest Elementary School by 1:00, but I can't use my car. What are some other things I can do to get there on time. I could call Therese and ask her to pick me up on her way to school. I could call Greg [his brother] and ask him to bring me my other set of car keys. I could break a car window and get my keys. I could just forget group and go back to the library. Let's see, Therese's car isn't running, and she wouldn't have it on campus anyway. Greg probably is home and could be

here in 15 minutes. If I break the window, it will cost me at least a hundred dollars. I have a lot of work to do, but the kids would be disappointed and hurt if I don't show up. I'll call Greg. So that's what I did.

In this example Eric modeled his thinking which happened to be a problem-solving sequence of thoughts. (Eric was studying Kendall & Braswell's [1985] book at the time.)

Subsequent to Eric's example, he and his co-therapist elicited the children's thoughts about the therapists not showing up on time. As the children expressed their thoughts, the therapists modeled more adaptive thoughts. Typically, the therapist models short coping statements that the child can use to control his or her symptoms. For example, "I woke up feeling kind of crummy so I thought: What can I do to help myself feel better? I could put on my favorite shirt, I'll eat lunch with Tom, and I'll play football after school even if I feel tired."

Problem-Solving Training

Training in problem solving serves a number of functions for depressed children. First, it counteracts the rigidity and narrow focus of their thinking. It helps them obtain a more flexible and broader perspective on things. Secondly, it provides the youths with a coping strategy that they may be lacking or using ineffectively. Depressed children, especially those who are suicidal, tend to be locked into one or a few ineffective coping strategies. They are not aware of alternative and potentially more effective procedures. Since the actions they try over and over again are ineffective, they develop a sense of hopelessness and futility. Problem solving helps empower them so that they feel as though they can take some actions to overcome their difficulties. Finally, as implied above, it provides children who are actually in a distressing situation with a method for helping themselves avoid, overcome, or lessen the impact of the situation. Thus, problem solving has both a cognitive and functional impact on the depressed youngster.

The problem-solving sequence that we have used is based on the sequence described by Meichenbaum (1977) and later by Kendall (e.g., 1981). The seven steps are outlined in Table 4.3. The first step of the procedure is problem definition. During this step, the child tries to identify and define the problem. For many children, this is a difficult process. Children often recognize that something is wrong or that they do not feel good, but they are unaware of what is causing

TABLE 4.3. Seven Steps of the Problem-Solving Sequence

Step	Content
1	Define the problem
2	Brainstorm to generate possible solutions
3	Focus attention and energy on the task
4	Project the outcome of each potential solution
5	Weigh the consequences and choose a solution
6	Evaluate the outcome of the chosen action
7	Self-reinforce for success or repeat the process of Steps 2–7

the problem or bad feelings. Thus, the child and therapist collaboratively proceed to identify the problems the child faces and the parameters of each problem. To some extent, being able to identify and place a label on a problem provides the child with some sense of relief. In some instances, the child has a multitude of problems. The therapist elicits the full gamut of problems and then prioritizes them with the child's input.

The second step of the process is the generation of possible solutions. This step is very difficult for depressed youngsters for a couple of reasons. Depressed children have a restricted and rigid approach to dealing with problems. In addition, because of their hopelessness, they tend to generate a minimum of possible solutions and tend to short-circuit the process early and give up. Finally, they often do not know many solutions because they have not had the necessary experiences.

Early in treatment, the therapist collaborates with the child to develop as many possible solutions to each problem. The child is taught that the key to success at this step is to not evaluate any of the solutions; rather, as many solutions as possible should be generated regardless of whether the child thinks they will work or not. The therapist commonly adds solutions to the child's list of possibilities.

During the third step, the child is taught to focus his or her attention on the task at hand. The objective of this phase is to help the child to muster his or her energy and to focus it on solving the problem.

The fourth step also appears to be a critical one. During the fourth step, the child is taught to project the outcomes of the proposed solutions. In other words, the therapist and child predict the possible outcomes of each proposed solution. During this process, the outcome of each possible solution is evaluated relative to the desired goal and the child's preferences. Once again, the therapist tends to be quite active in the process, often helping the child to see what the possible outcomes would be.

The fifth step is to review the possible solutions and choose one. Once a solution is chosen, the child enacts the planned solution.

The sixth step is to evaluate the outcome of the chosen solution and to compare it to the desired goal. If the outcome is acceptable, the child self-rewards (Step 7) for doing a good job. If the outcome is unacceptable, the child considers the information while selecting another possible solution, and the last four steps are repeated.

The problem-solving steps are taught to the children through a number of procedures. Typically the process has to be directly taught to the children. This is accomplished through self-instructional training that is described in the following section. In addition, a number of somewhat less direct procedures are used, including cognitive modeling and brainstorming. As noted in the previous section, the therapist can think aloud whenever he or she faces a problem during the sessions, or, when the child faces a problem, the therapist can model the thoughts that the child might follow to solve the problem. A frequently used procedure is for the child and therapist to identify problems that the child is facing. After identifying a problem, the child and therapist brainstorm and talk through the problem-solving steps. The therapist is continually vigilant for opportunities to do this. Each time the child and therapist do this, the therapist tries to ask more questions and give fewer answers to help the child actively think his or her way through it.

Self-Instructional Training

Self-instructional training is a therapeutic procedure that can be used to help a child internalize a set of self-statements that can be used to guide the child's behavior or thinking. The training procedure that we have used was originally developed by Meichenbaum and Goodman (1971) and later modified by Kendall (e.g., 1977). An outline of this procedure can be found in Table 4.4. The content of the thoughts that are taught through the training can be anything. For example, the child can be taught to say: "Remember, they are not making fun of you; they are just fooling around. They do that to everyone." Similarly, the child can be taught a set of self-instructions that guide him or her through the problem-solving process.

A child may be taught to think of the following self-statements that guide the problem-solving process:

1. What's the problem?
2. Think of all of the possibilities.

3. Clear my head, relax, and concentrate.
4. What would happen if?
5. Choose the best one.
6. How did I do?
7. I did a good job.
   I made a mistake so I'll start over.

TABLE 4.4. Self-Instructional Training Sequence

1. The child watches as the therapist talks aloud while completing a task.
2. The child performs the task while instructing him- or herself out loud.
3. The child watches as the therapist whispers self-guiding directions while completing the task.
4. The child watches as the therapist completes the task and gives behavioral indications of using self-instructions.
5. The child completes the task using covert self-instructions.

Note. Adapted from Kendall (1977).

This set of self-statements matches the seven steps of the problem-solving process, and they can be taught to the child through self-instructional training. The medium that can be used to teach the self-statements can be of a personal nature, or it can be made more fun by playing a game. Kendall (1981) notes that using a game helps remove some of the emotionality from the learning experience, which may facilitate learning. Thus, we commonly begin by using a board game such as checkers, Chinese checkers, or Othello. These games provide the child with immediate feedback for when he or she fails to use his or her self-instructions correctly (e.g., the child loses a chip).

Prior to starting the game, the therapist checks with the child to be sure that he or she understands the rules of the game. Then, the self-instructions are introduced as a strategy that the child can use to play better. First the therapist models the use of the self-instructions and what they actually mean. The child is queried to ensure that he or she truly understands what is meant by each of the seven statements. Then the therapist asks the child to write each of the statements down in his or her own words on a 3-by-5 card. The child can use this card as a prompt whenever it is his or her turn. Then the child performs the task while saying aloud each of the statements and giving verbal and behavioral cues that he or she is actually trying to follow the statements. Next the therapist takes a turn and once again models the self-statements by saying them aloud as he or she takes a turn. This process continues until the child clearly understands how to use the self-statements and is beginning to demonstrate that they are becoming internalized. At this point, the therapist begins the fading process by whispering the self-statements, and the child may also be asked to whisper them as he or she uses them. As further evidence of mastery accrues, the therapist switches to covert self-guidance followed by the child switching to covert self-guidance. As the sessions progress, whenever the child makes a mistake during a game, the therapist instructs the child to switch back to overtly stating the self-instructions as a check to ensure that he or she is still using them correctly.

After the child has mastered the self-statements, the therapist begins asking the child how he or she would use them to solve everyday personal problems. Once again, the therapist might begin by modeling the overt use of the self-instructions and then work through the rest of the steps of the training process with the child.

5

Self-Control, Behavioral, and Family Treatment Procedures

In Chapter 4 some of the more useful cognitive restructuring procedures were described, and it was noted that it is often necessary to delay the implementation of these procedures until after the child has gained some control over his or her depressive symptoms and some distance from his or her depressogenic thinking. Both of these objectives are achieved through the use of self-control and more traditional behavioral procedures. There is another overriding objective of using the behavioral procedures; it is changing the child's thinking about him- or herself, his or her sense of self-efficacy, and other relevant thoughts.

SELF-CONTROL PROCEDURES

Rehm (1977) has developed a model of depression that is based on the thesis that depression results from deficits in self-control skills. More specifically, Rehm hypothesizes that depressed individuals (1) self-monitor the negative events in their lives to the exclusion of the positive events, (2) set excessively stringent standards for their performance and as a consequence are unable to achieve such standards, (3) make internal attributions for their failures and external attributions for their successes, and (4) tend to self-punish more and self-reinforce less than their nondepressed peers. There is some empirical support for these deficits existing in depressed children (Kaslow et al., 1984). In addition, Seligman et al. (1984) reported support for the belief that an insidious attributional style was associated with depression in children. Our own research (see Kendall et al., 1989) supports the notion that depressed children evaluate themselves significantly more negatively than do nondepressed children; however, this is not the result of setting excessively stringent standards for their performance. In fact, there was no difference in the standards set by depressed and nondepressed youths across the three studies we completed. Nonetheless, depressed children evaluate themselves more negatively than nondepressed children.

Rehm (e.g., Fuchs & Rehm, 1977; Rehm et al., 1987) has developed a treatment program that is designed to remediate these deficits, and this program has been adapted (Stark et al., 1987) for moderately depressed school children (see Chapter 2). The training procedure used to teach children self-control skills for coping with their depressive symptoms is described in the following sections of this chapter. However, at this time, self-control procedures comprise just one portion of the treatment program. Other cognitive and behavioral procedures also seem to be necessary for successful treatment.

Self-Monitoring

Self-monitoring is the conscious act of observing one's own thoughts, feelings, overt behavior, or more private physical reactions (e.g., increased heart rate, muscle tension) and making a judgment about their occurrence or nonoccurrence. After making a judgment about the occurrence or nonoccurrence of one of these target responses, the child records this information in some manner. A youngster also might be asked to self-monitor other information that is relevant to a particular thought, behavior, or emotion. For example, the child may be asked to observe the situation he or she is in when feelings of sadness become apparent. The child also may be asked to observe and note who else is there and what they are doing. Thus, self-monitoring is a purposeful and conscious act of observing oneself and the situations one enters. The second step is to indicate the outcome of the self-observation through some permanent recording procedure such as through placing slash marks on a sheet of paper after each time the child talks with a peer.

When treating depressed children, self-monitoring is used as both an assessment tool and a treatment procedure. It may in fact be difficult to disentangle these two uses, since self-observation can in and of itself lead to change in some individuals. However, for the sake of clarity, a distinction will be drawn. When self-monitoring is used as an assessment procedure, the goal is to have the child gather therapeutically relevant information. When self-monitoring is used as a treatment technique, it is used as a way to redirect the child's attention in a more therapeutically relevant, adaptive fashion and as a means of guiding the implementation of other treatment procedures. As an assessment tool, self-monitoring is used to gather information about (1) the child's overt and covert worlds, (2) activities that the child enjoys and that elevate his or her mood, (3) the implementation of new skills, and (4) cognitions that may lead to various depressive symptoms. As a treatment procedure, self-monitoring is used to (1) change the child's focus from the negative events occurring in his or her life to the positive events, (2) document improvement in symptomatology that results from using new skills, and (3) identify depressogenic cognitions and guide their replacement with more adaptive thoughts through the use of cognitive restructuring.

Self-Monitoring as an Assessment Tool

Understanding the Child. In its role as an assessment device, self-monitoring may be the first therapeutic tool used. It also is an assessment procedure that is used throughout treatment. Initially, self-monitoring is used as an adjunctive procedure to the interview for acquiring information about the child's life situation and his or her way of constructing it. The information that is acquired through self-monitoring is used by the therapist as a means of concretizing and personalizing the therapeutic rationale imparted during affective education (see Chapter 4). The therapist illustrates the relationship among thoughts, feelings, and behaviors through examples provided from the child's self-monitoring records.

Information acquired through self-monitoring helps the therapist understand the context in which the child lives. As such, it helps the therapist identify stressors in the child's life. This is an important therapeutic function, since the author's research (e.g., Best & Stark, 1990) indicates that depressed children, relative to nondepressed children, experience significantly more stressful events in their lives. Especially problematic are chronic stressors such as living with a chronically ill parent. A partial list of the chronic stressors, major life events, and daily hassles that are associated with depression among children are reported in Tables 5.1, 5.2, and 5.3, respectively, and a discussion of procedures for helping the child cope with these stressors appears in a later portion of this chapter.

Children often are vague in their descriptions of things that bother

TABLE 5.1. Examples of Chronic Strains That Are Associated with Depression

Personal illnesses	*Home environment*
Allergies	Messy
Asthma	Dirty
Frequent headaches	Dark
Serious physical problems	Noisy
Parent's or sibling's illnesses	*School environment*
Anemia	Teacher expects too much
Asthma	Other students laugh at my
Heart trouble	mistakes
Serious back trouble	Smart students get more
Cancer	privileges
Emotional problems	

them. Self-monitoring can be used as a means of acquiring specific information that fleshes out the child's initial report. For example, during the initial interview the youngster may not be clear about what his parents do to "criticize" him, yet he feels as though they do it a lot. In such a case, the child would be instructed to monitor his feelings and to note what is happening every time he feels as though he is being criticized over the following week. Immediately after his parents are finished talking to him, he records in a narrative form what was happening, what preceded the criticism, who was doing

TABLE 5.2. Examples of Major Life Events That Are Associated with Depression

The death of a parent

Marital separation of your parents

Remarriage of a parent to a step-parent

Birth of a brother or sister

Hospitalization of a brother or sister

Loss of a job by your mother or father

Major increase or decrease in your parents' income

A new adult moving into your home

Move to a new school district

Failing a grade in school

TABLE 5.3. Examples of Daily Hassles That
Are Associated with Depression

Fighting or arguing with someone

Being yelled at, scolded, or criticized

Being punished

Losing a game or race

Being left out, rejected, or ignored

Doing poorly at school (see, failing a test)

Breaking or losing something

Doing something bad

Missing someone (friend, parent)

Not being able to do something you want to do

---

the criticizing, and what was said. Similarly, a child might report that she is being "punished all of the time." In this case, the child might be asked to keep track of each time that she is punished over the ensuing week. In addition, the child would be asked to note what happened before she was punished and the extent of the punishment levied.

Information obtained through self-monitoring guides treatment. Such information might indicate that an environmental intervention is needed or that the family might benefit from some form of therapy. However, given the depressed child's tendency to distort information, it is important to corroborate the youngster's reports with information gathered from siblings, parents, and other knowledgeable people. This information also is used as an aid to the therapist when cognitive restructuring is used. For example, the child may feel as though his parents do not like him and offer the facts that they criticize and punish him a lot. Since the child collected information that verifies this fact, the therapist might identify other evidence that verifies that the parents like him (if this is in fact the case) or alternative means of interpreting the parents' behavior that allow the child to still feel like a worthwhile person. Of equal importance, if this information is true, then the therapist would concurrently work with the child's parents to change their behavior as well as the reciprocal pattern of behaviors exhibited by the child and parents that leads up to and includes the actual criticism and punishment.

Assessment of Treatment Effectiveness. As the child client is taught skills for controlling his or her depressive symptoms, he or she is asked to self-monitor their use and effectiveness. The objective of this self-monitoring is twofold. First, it serves as a means of assessing whether the child is following the correct steps for implementing the skill and for identifying unforeseen impediments to using the skill correctly. Second, by having the child consciously note his or her successful use of the skills, the child gains a sense of self-efficacy. Thus, self-monitoring of the use of coping skills serves in part as a means of troubleshooting. The information helps the therapist correct the way the child implements and uses a particular coping skill. This is an ongoing process that leads the therapist to do some additional training when needed. Whenever a new skill is taught during a session, the child is asked to self-monitor his or her *in vivo* use of the skill as an implementation check.

Implementation Issues. When using self-monitoring as an assessment procedure, the child is taught to use a procedure that varies along a continuum of how structured it is. At the unstructured end of the continuum, the therapist instructs the child to note mentally and record the occurrence of specified events. At the structured end, the approach involves instructing the child to use preconstructed self-monitoring sheets. For example, to gain an understanding of what is going on in the child's life, lists of pleasant and unpleasant things that happen, of things that one thinks about, and of things that one does are typed on a sheet of paper. The lists include a number of blank spaces that the child can use to record events that are not already included. These self-monitoring records are commonly referred to as pleasant and unpleasant events schedules. Examples of a pleasant and unpleasant events, schedules for fourth, fifth, and sixth graders can be found in Appendices F, G, and H, respectively.

When instructing the child to self-monitor, it is necessary to make the directions as concrete and specific as possible. This is a collaborative process that involves the child. The first step in the training procedure is to explain to the child the value of completing the self-monitoring. The rationale should be specific to the child and the procedure to be employed. The second step is defining the event to be monitored. It is imperative that the child clearly understands what he or she is supposed to be self-monitoring prior to asking the child to do it. The therapist should offer examples, and then the child should be asked to provide his or her own examples. When a more structured procedure is used that involves a preconstructed self-monitoring sheet, it is important for the child to understand what each behavior on the sheet means. The third step is to describe the procedure the child will follow to record the necessary information. For example, "right after you've been punished you will get your notebook and note what day it is, what happened, who punished you, and what the punishment was. You'll write these things down as soon as possible after they happen." With an unstructured approach, the child may be asked to write down in a narrative fashion the information that is being self-monitored. The child needs to know where to record the information as well as what to record. Typically, this information is recorded in a notebook. It is helpful to have the child maintain the recordings in one place where they will not get lost and where they can be kept in chronological order.

A critical point to be emphasized with the child is the importance of self-recording *immediately* after the specified event has occurred. A delay in time can lead to a distortion resulting from reliance on memory or to the child's forgetting to record the event altogether. Experience with the more structured approach suggests that it may be more prone to the children delaying the recording of the event. Since the children simply have to check off what was happening, they commonly think that they can remember what they are supposed to record and put off until later the act of self-recording.

It is useful to brainstorm with the child in an attempt to identify potential impediments to completing the self-monitoring assignment successfully. Typically, this involves asking the child what he or she would do if any number of potential impediments occurred. For example, "What could you do if you forgot your notebook at school and you needed to record an incident of criticism?" "What are you going to do if you have just been criticized, and your parents tell you to go and clean your room?" The child should be encouraged to contribute to this process, since he or she commonly has greater foresight into potential roadblocks than the therapist. After a roadblock has been identified, the therapist and child develop a plan for avoiding or overcoming the roadblock should it occur.

The final step in the self-monitoring training process is to review the self-monitoring assignment with the child prior to sending him or her off to do it. The key components of the assignment are reviewed including (1) what will be monitored, (2) how it will be recorded, (3) when and how often it will be recorded, and (4) what the child will do if a variety of potential problems should arise.

The process of teaching a child to self-monitor is an ongoing one. Like any skill, the child gets better at it with practice. The therapist needs to review with the child his or her efforts at self-monitoring on a regular basis. Not only does it provide the therapist with useful information, but it serves as a source of reinforcement for completing the assignment. At the beginning of each session the therapist commonly reviews the child's efforts as well as the results of the self-monitoring. Any problems completing the assignment are dealt with in a collaborative, problem-to-be-solved fashion with the objective being more accurate, precise, and timely self-monitoring.

Monitoring Pleasant Events. A procedure that has been borrowed from the adult treatment literature is self-monitoring of engagement in pleasant events. The term pleasant events is somewhat of a misnomer, since the individual self-monitors more than just the enjoyable things that happen in his or her life. Typically, the client also monitors the positive thoughts that he or she has as well as pleasant activities that he or she engages in. It is this latter focus that may be the key, since it leads to increased involvement in pleasant activities. In the pleasant events schedules that we have developed for children, the number of positive things that happen in the child's life has been expanded relative to the schedules that typically are used with adults. This was done purposely to reflect the fact that children have less control over their lives relative to adults. Thus, they are somewhat more at the mercy of their environments. So an attempt was made to capture this developmental difference in these pleasant events schedules. Examples of the schedules can be found in Appendices F, G, and H.

1. Construction of Pleasant Events Schedules. The schedules that are found in the appendices were empirically derived. At this time they may be somewhat dated, since children's activities are driven by fads. Thus, it would be useful to update such lists continually. The following procedure was used to identify the items that comprise the schedule. A form with five lines on it followed by three smiley faces was developed. A copy of this form can be found in Appendix I. The children were instructed to think about and come up with a list of the five things they enjoy doing the most. After writing down their answers, they were instructed to place an X over the smiley face that best illustrated how much fun the activity is. Similar assessment forms were developed for identifying pleasant thoughts and things that happen to children. The same procedure was followed by the children to complete these latter two forms. Once a number of children from each grade level ($n = 100$) had completed the forms, the forms were scored, and the activities, thoughts, and events were rank ordered according to how frequently each thing was listed and by its position in the child's list (e.g, first vs. fifth). Finally, only activities, thoughts, or events that had a positive smiley face rating were included. Individual pleasant events schedules were developed for each grade.

As the reader will notice, at the bottom of the pleasant events schedule is an 11-point Likert-type scale. This scale is used by the children as a means of rating their mood each day. At the end of the day, the child completes the mood rating according to how he or she felt in general over that day.

2. Implementation Issues. The training procedure used to teach children how to use the pleasant events schedules is relatively simple and consists of the steps noted above for training self-monitoring in general. There are a few additions to this procedure that have been used when working with groups of children. After the children have been (1) reminded of the three things that contribute to their mood (what they do and think, and things that happen in their lives), (2) given a rationale for the self-monitoring, and (3) instructed what and how to self-monitor, they play a game designed to provide them with some practice at completing the pleasant events schedules.

Prior to the session, the therapist writes down each item from the pleasant events schedule on a separate 3 × 5 card. A few cards with negative events and a number of cards with positive events not included on the schedule are added to the deck. The deck is placed in the middle of the table, and each child is given a pleasant events schedule. Then, each takes turns drawing a card from the deck and reading it aloud. The therapist facilitates a discussion about when the children last engaged in the activity and what it felt like to do it. After picking a card, the child locates the item on the pleasant events schedule and places a check mark on the line that precedes the item. If a pleasant event is picked that is not on the schedule form, then the child writes it down in one of the blank spaces. The therapist coaches the children through the game and encourages the children to help one another. After all of the cards have been picked, the children take turns reviewing their hand of cards, and then they rate what they think their mood would be for that day if those things had really happened. The other children and therapist provide each child with feedback about his or her overall mood rating.

After the game is over and all questions have been answered, the children are given enough copies of the pleasant events schedules so that they have one for each day that will pass between sessions. In addition, the children write the days of the week across the top of the schedules so that they can be kept in chronological order. Finally each child is given a 3-ring binder, and the schedules are placed in it.

The children are instructed to complete the forms, which involves placing a check mark in front of each item that occurs on that day, a minimum of three times per day including once right after lunch break and recess, right before leaving for home, and finally right before going to bed. During this last time the child also completes the mood rating. Subsequently, the children generate possible impediments to completing the task, and the group helps each child develop plans for overcoming the problems.

Results of this self-monitoring serve a number of therapeutic functions that are discussed in the following section. They also serve the assessment function of helping the therapist identify activities, thoughts, and events that are associated with elevated mood. To accomplish this, the therapist graphs the number of pleasant events the child recorded and the child's mood rating. A copy of this graph paper can be found in Appendix J. The therapist completes the graphing between sessions but discusses the results with the child. With older and brighter clients, the child completes the graph with some help from the therapist. Patterns in the child's graph are identified by the child and therapist. Of relevance to the assessment of pleasant activities are patterns that suggest that a specific activity is associated with elevated mood. For example, every time a boy goes to the go-cart track, he rates his mood for the day an 8, which is almost twice his mood rating on other days.

Self-Monitoring as a Treatment Tool

As a treatment procedure, self-monitoring of pleasant events serves as a means of focusing the child's attention on more positive things. Depressed children tend to notice the negative things going on in their lives and overlook the positive things. By getting the child consciously to direct his or her attention to the pleasant things he or she does, thinks, and has happen, the negative cycle is interrupted. In addition, it may lead to some cognitive restructuring as the child consciously watches for and records positive information. The child's schema of the world being a place filled with personally detracting experiences may be altered as the youngster collects information that provides contradictory evidence.

Self-monitoring of engagement in pleasant activities oftentimes leads to another positive therapeutic outcome: The child begins to do more fun things, which leads to an improvement in mood, which leads to the child being more active, and so forth. Some children turn this into a game. They see a challenge to trying to do more fun things each day. This seems to lead to a positive snowballing effect in which the children do more and more enjoyable activities. The information about pleasant activities is used in the activity-scheduling procedure to be described later.

Results of the mood and activity graph contribute to a sense of self-efficacy as the child sees concrete evidence that he or she can control emotions through engagement in pleasant activities. Over time, a gradual increase in mood becomes evident and is sustained. Similarly, as the child self-monitors the use of other coping skills and the resultant improvement in mood, the child's sense of self-efficacy is further enhanced.

Commonly, depressed children only partially complete their self-monitoring assignment. This partial failure can confirm a negative self-evaluation (e.g., "I can't do anything right"). Thus, it is important for the child to experience a sense of success for putting forth some effort and at least trying to self-monitor. This places the therapist in a difficult position, since successful treatment is based in part on the child's self-monitoring. The therapist walks a fine line between being overly demanding, which leads to failure, and continually allowing the child to fail to complete the self-monitoring necessary for change to occur. It is important to identify the point where the child completes as much self-monitoring as possible while not placing the child in a spot where he or she will definitely fail.

A number of procedures have been used to motivate the youngster to follow the self-monitoring instructions as closely as possible. One procedure is behavioral contracting. A sample contract can be found in Appendix K. This contract is altered to include additional information when it is used to increase the probability of completing self-monitoring. Specifically, the contract should state what is expected of the child and what the therapist will do in return. What the child is being asked to monitor, how he or she will self-record, and how often he or she will self-monitor are clearly stated in the contract. The therapists' part of the contract usually is to reward the child in some way that is clearly stated in the contract. Once the contingencies have been spelled out, the child and the therapist sign the contract. It is critical for the therapist to honor his or her end of the contract. If the child does not fulfill his or her portion of the agreement, then the therapist should withhold the reward. When this occurs, the child and therapist work together to develop a plan to ensure success the next time the child is asked to self-monitor.

When the youngster's parents are healthy and there is a productive relationship between the child and parents, the parents may be asked to help the child remember to complete the self-monitoring. The parents are instructed gently to remind the child to complete the self-monitoring. They are specifically instructed not to let their reminders become a point of argument. In addition, the parents are taught to emphasize success and to be encouraging rather than punishing. Punishment and criticism are emphatically discouraged.

Self-Evaluation Training

Negative self-evaluation is one of the cardinal symptoms of depressed children (Kendall et al., 1989). Although Rehm (1977) originally hypothesized that depressed individuals negatively evaluate their performance because they set excessively stringent standards for their performance that they cannot achieve, our research indicates that all children set relatively high standards of performance. The difference between depressed and nondepressed children is the way in which they evaluate themselves. Depressed children simply evaluate their performances, possessions, and personal qualities more negatively.

Self-evaluation training is an integral component of self-control treatments for depressed adults (e.g., Rehm et al., 1987) and depressed children (Stark et al., 1987). It also is one of the components of the treatment program we have developed for depressed children. Traditionally in the literature, self-evaluation training has been used with children who have behavioral disorders. It was used as an adjunctive procedure to more traditional behavioral techniques such as a token economy. The hope was that the addition of self-evaluation training would lead to greater maintenance-of-treatment effects. In fact, there is some evidence to support this contention (e.g., Drabman, Spitalnik, & O'Leary, 1973; Kaufman & O'Leary, 1972; Turkewitz, O'Leary, & Ironsmith, 1975). It is important to note that the objectives of this treatment component and the procedure that is followed when implementing it are different when it is being used with depressed children as compared to when it is being used with children who are experiencing externalizing disorders.

To date, it appears as though most of the empirically evaluated self-evaluation training procedures for children have been based on a deficit model (e.g., Kendall & Braswell, 1985). It has been assumed that children lack self-evaluation skills, that they do not pay attention to their performance and consciously evaluate it. This may in fact be the case with children who have other disorders; however, depressed children are very conscious of their performance and their evaluations of it. Their problem appears to be one of distortion. They are overly negative in their self-evaluations. Thus, the focus of treatment is on changing the distortion or *how* they evaluate it, rather than teaching them to be more aware of their behavior and *to* evaluate it.

There are two primary objectives to the self-evaluation training procedure. The first objective is to teach the child to evaluate him- or herself less harshly. The second objective is to identify areas of importance to the child, where he or she negatively evaluates him- or herself and is objectively deficient, and then to teach the child skills that will lead to self-improvement. As presently conceived, self-evaluation training is a specific case of cognitive restructuring. The therapist helps the youngster learn how to evaluate him- or herself more realistically and rationally. For many children, this means helping them to use the same criteria for evaluating their own performance that they use when evaluating the performance of others. Many times the children are much harder on themselves than they are on others. It also involves helping them to recognize their positive attributes, outcomes, and possessions. Many of the previously described cognitive restructuring procedures and self-monitoring are used during this training.

One of the difficulties the therapist faces is determining when the child is striving for excellence and when the child's strivings become debilitating. As a society we emphasize achievement, and our children receive a lot of messages about the need to perform. Commonly their parents have high expectations for them (Adam & Stark, 1990). It can be quite unacceptable to a set of parents to learn that the therapist is going to help their child learn how not to push him- or herself so hard in school. In fact, some children have been denied access to treatment or declined treatment because it would take away from their time in class or their study time. When we have checked their GPA, they were extremely high achievers.

Phase I: Identification and Modification of Standards and Self-Evaluations

A multiphase training procedure is used to teach children a more adaptive means of self-evaluation. The first phase involves the assessment of the child's standards and self-evaluations. This is accomplished in a number of ways. The first way is to be alert during the interview so as to note the child's revelations of his or her self-evaluations through spontaneous statements. For example, the child might say "I'm no good at school stuff." Similarly, a negative self-evaluation may underlie a statement such as "I'll never have a girlfriend." Underlying this statement is the self-evaluation of "I'm ugly and unlovable." The pervasiveness of such comments can serve as a rough gauge of the severity of the problem. At any point in time, given the considerations noted in Chapter 4, the therapist may choose to intervene by using a cognitive restructuring procedure. When it is a serious problem, which is typical of depressed youths, then it may be necessary to devote a number of sessions specifically to self-evaluation training.

A more formal and structured approach can be used to assess the youngster's self-evaluations. This can be accomplished by administering the My Standards Questionnaire, which can be found in Appendix L. This questionnaire, which has been surprisingly useful, has evolved over the years from an activity that was used as a brief treatment activity to an assessment device that provides the clinician with a lot of useful information. The questionnaire consists of four sections that provide the examiner with an indication of the child's perceptions of the standards his or her parents hold for him or her, the child's self-imposed standards, the child's self-evaluations, and a rank ordering of the value of each area that has been assessed. The 10 areas that the child evaluates him- or herself in were empirically derived through a nomination procedure. The 10 most frequently nominated areas were included in the questionnaire.

The questionnaire yields three scores and two difference scores. The scores include a total score for the parents' standards, the child's standards, and the child's overall self-evaluation. These scores are computed by summing the child's ratings across the 10 items that comprise each of the three sections. The two difference scores are computed by subtracting the child's overall self-evaluation from his or her parents' standards and then from his or her own standards. The latter difference score provides the clinician with an indication of whether the child is exceeding (a negatively valued number), meeting (a total score at or close to 0), or failing to meet his or her standards (a positively valenced number). The larger the difference score, the more positively or negatively the child is evaluating him- or herself. The difference score that is based on perceived parental standards can be interpreted in a similar fashion. Comparison of standards and self-evaluations on individual items enables the therapist to identify specific areas of perceived strength and weakness. This information is used as a guide for developing plans for self-improvement.

After the child has completed the questionnaire, he or she can assist in the scoring process, which helps illustrate for the child his or her standards and self-evaluations. The child can explain why he or she endorsed a given rating. This is a particularly useful group activity. Other group members can provide the youngster with feedback. However, the therapist has to be on his or her toes, since children do not live by the adage of "If you don't have anything nice to say, don't say anything at all." Rather, their feedback can be quite critical.

Sometimes, these children will endorse perfectionistic standards for themselves. In such instances it is important to use a vertical approach to assessment (see Chapter 4) and identify what it means for the child to obtain, or fail to obtain, that standard. Subsequently, the rationality of the standard and the meaning of it for the child can be discussed.

Once the irrationality or the maladaptivity of the standard has been illustrated, cognitive restructuring procedures can be used to help the child give up the standard. Subsequently, the therapist and child work together to establish more adaptive and realistic standards. For example, "It would be nice to look like Christie Brinkley, but I can feel good about myself by just looking the best that I can." The emotional value of setting more adaptive standards can be illustrated by asking the child to think about the old standard and own it, and experience how it feels to own that standard. Then the child is asked to think about and take ownership of the new, more adaptive standard and experience how it feels to own it.

When the child sets realistic and adaptive standards, but the child evaluates him- or herself negatively, a somewhat different procedure is followed. In this case, cognitive restructuring procedures and self-monitoring are used to help the child evaluate him- or herself in a more adaptive fashion. For example, let us consider the case of the child who would be satisfied if she was of average or a bit above average appearance but who thinks she is ugly. The first consideration is to assess the situation objectively to determine whether the child's self-evaluation of "I'm ugly" is accurate. If it is, then a vertical assessment is in order, and the therapist would try to determine whether the child is placing extreme and unreasonable meaning in being physically unattractive. If so, then this would be the focus of intervention. Also, if it is true, the therapist and child could work together to develop plans for self-improvement. This will be discussed below.

If the child's self-evaluation is unrealistic, which is the case with most depressed children, then the therapist would use "What's the evidence." The therapist and child would gather and explore the evidence that supports and disputes the self-evaluation. The therapist also might choose to use cognitive modeling and demonstrate for the child a more reasonable self-evaluation. In most cases, both procedures would be used. First, "What's the evidence" would be used to help discredit the existing self-evaluation, and then, as the youngster began to question his or her self-evaluation, the therapist would model a more realistic and adaptive self-evaluation. As the therapist models the new self-evaluation, he or she reviews the evidence that supports the new self-evaluation.

To help solidify the new self-evaluation, the youngster would be instructed to self-monitor the evidence that supports it. Over the course of a number of sessions, the therapist and child would review the evidence that supports the new self-evaluation. As the child begins to incorporate the new self-evaluation, the therapist checks with the child to find out how the change in self-evaluation has affected the child's emotional state.

The next step is to identify additional areas where the child negatively evaluates him- or herself. Once these are identified, the therapist encourages the child to apply cognitive restructuring and self-monitoring to modify other maladaptive self-evaluations. The therapist models and coaches the child through the process.

Phase II: Working toward Self-Improvement

The second phase of self-evaluation training involves teaching the child to translate personal standards into realistic goals and then to develop and carry out a plan for attaining the goals. During the first phase, areas where the child is not living up to his or her standards are identified. When it is reasonable for the child to hold the standard, and when it would be advantageous to achieve the standard, then the therapist and child clearly define the standard; for example, I want to eliminate my pimples and consistently bathe, which includes washing my hair.

The next step is to prioritize the areas of desired change. It is important for the therapist to encourage the child to choose a goal to begin working on that is relatively easy to achieve. This goal might not be the highest-priority goal, but success in this endeavor is of primary importance. Once the goal has been chosen, the therapist and child collaboratively develop a plan to obtain it.

Problem solving is used as the means of developing the plan. If possible, the goal is broken down into subgoals. Brainstorming is used to develop plans for obtaining each subgoal and eventually the goal. After generating all possible actions that could be followed to achieve the goal, the therapist and child project the potential outcome of each action. After completing this process, the child chooses the actions that are most likely to lead to the successful completion of the plan.

To further insure the success of the plan, after it has been formulated, the therapist and child try to generate possible impediments to successfully carrying it out. As each possible roadblock is identified, the therapist and child generate plans for overcoming the impediment.

Once the plan has been established, the child is instructed to self-monitor his or her progress carrying out the plan and achieving subgoals. The child and therapist review the child's progress and revise the plans as necessary.

Self-Reinforcement Training

Self-reinforcement is the process of presenting rewards to oneself contingent on desired performance. Self-reinforcement training is a component of a self-control treatment program for depressed adults (e.g., Rehm et al., 1987), adolescents (Reynolds & Coats, 1986), and children (Stark et al., 1987). It may be one of the most effective treatment procedures with a variety of behavior disorders (O'Leary & Dubey, 1979). Self-reinforcement has the same impact on behavior as externally administered rewards. It leads to an increase in the probability that the behavior will recur in the future. It often serves as a bridge between acquiring and utilizing new skills and the resultant improvement in symptomatology.

Although self-reinforcement is used in a variety of ways during treatment, its primary use is to increase the probability that the client will enact a particular behavior. The child is taught to self-reinforce whenever he or she tries to complete a therapeutic homework assignment or to use one of the therapeutic procedures. It is hoped that this self-reinforcement will lead to an increase in the use of these coping skills.

The idea of reinforcing oneself is quite foreign to depressed children. From my experience in treating children with a variety of disorders, it seems as though depressed children have much more trouble learning how to self-reinforce, and they experience more difficulty with actually reinforcing themselves. They do not seem to understand that it is okay to reinforce oneself. Thus, often it is necessary for the therapist to identify the beliefs that underlie the youngster's reluctance to self-reinforce. Then, cognitive restructuring procedures (see Chapter 4) would be used to alter these beliefs.

Once again, a multiphase training program is used to teach the child how to self-reinforce. The first phase of the training procedure is to identify potential rewards. Whereas this is easy to do with nondepressed children, it is difficult to do with depressed children. Because of the symptom of anhedonia, they do not derive pleasure from previously enjoyed activities. Thus, few things are rewarding. Nonetheless, the therapist assesses possible rewards. An initial assessment can be made using the questionnaire found in Appendix M. If the child reported that nothing was rewarding anymore, then, the child would be asked to complete it as he or she would have prior to the onset of the episode of depression. Some children can do this, whereas others cannot change to this alternative time frame.

Since the child may have difficulty remembering rewards, it may be necessary to involve the child's parents in the assessment process. They are interviewed to identify objects, events, activities, and thoughts that are or were rewarding for the child. After the possible rewards have been identified, the therapist determines the availability of the rewards for the child. Since the parents often are in control of access to these rewards, it is imperative that the parents participate in this process. Once available rewards have been identified, the therapist interviews the child to determine the desirability of each reward. Thus, the most potent rewards are identified.

A potentially limiting factor in self-reinforcement training with children is the fact that they have significantly less control over their lives. This is equally true of the minimal control they have over the self-administration of rewards. Children often do not have the financial means to purchase material rewards or to pay for many of the activities that are rewarding to them. Even if they have the money they need, they may be dependent on an adult for transportation that is necessary to obtain the reward. At a more basic level, children often need their parents' permission to make a purchase or to do something. Thus, parental support often is a prerequisite to self-reinforcement by a child.

In an attempt to recognize and deal with the dependence on parental support, it is common practice for the therapist to solicit the parents' support. The therapist works with the depressed child's parents to get an agreement from them to try, within reasonable limits, to provide their youngster with greater access to desired rewards of a material and activity nature. The concept of reinforcement is explained to the parents, and their concerns are discussed. Since the child's parents have been involved in the assessment process, they are reminded of the rewards their child might desire. In addition, they are informed of the types of things the child will be doing to earn the reward. A common concern of the parents is that the child will abuse the self-reinforcement by being overly liberal in the self-administration. Experience and research (e.g., Bandura & Perloff, 1967) indicate that children in general are conservative in their self-administration of rewards. Depressed children are especially restrictive in self-reinforcement. With such youngsters, it would be preferable for them to err on the side of being overly generous.

As parental support is being secured, the therapist teaches the child the principles of reinforcement including the impact of rewards, importance of contingent administration of rewards, and the administration of rewards of parallel value to the difficulty of the task. A lengthy education process is followed to accomplish this goal.

The first step in the training phase is to define reinforcement and punishment. Consistent with the overall approach to therapy, the child is not told what these constructs are; rather, the child is queried and encouraged to participate in defining them through personal examples. The impact of reinforcement and punishment on behavior can be illustrated through a common experience, such as training a pet to do tricks. Many children are familiar with this. It also serves as a good illustration of the importance of immediacy and continuous schedules of reinforcement.

When children think of rewards, they usually think of just one class of rewards: material rewards, especially treats such as soda, ice cream, or a favorite snack. It is necessary to introduce the children to other classes of rewards including pleasant activities and positive thoughts. The positive emotional impact of both of these classes of rewards is emphasized, as well as their everyday, normal use.

For self-reinforcement to have the desired impact on behavior, rewards must be administered contingent on enactment of specific behaviors. The concept of contingent administration of rewards is illustrated through the child's own everyday examples as well as through questions that illustrate the importance of contingent self-reinforcement in the training of a pet. However, depressed children also are encouraged to self-reinforce just for the "fun of it" because of the uplifting positive impact it has.

The client is taught that rewards vary along a continuum of how potent they are. Their potency is gauged by how much enjoyment is derived from them. The child is asked to take his or her list of rewards and to prioritize them according to their degree of enjoyment. After the rewards have been rank-ordered, the child is taught to use large rewards to reinforce him- or herself for completion of difficult or demanding tasks, medium rewards for moderate tasks, and less valuable rewards for easy or simple tasks. In addition, the child is taught to administer the lesser rewards for completion of small portions of a large task.

Finally, the motivational utility of imaging rewards during task completion is discussed. The child is taught to imagine the larger more valued reward while completing a difficult or demanding task. The image can have a motivating effect on the child that can lead to task persistence. In conjunction with the imagery, the child is encouraged to self-reinforce with less valued rewards.

The education process typically takes four to six sessions. Before the child is instructed to self-reinforce outside of the sessions, the therapist models the process for the child through hypothetical examples. In addition, the therapist and child try to identify possible impediments to the successful implementation of self-reinforcement. As the possible roadblocks are identified, the child and therapist use problem solving to develop plans for overcoming them.

BEHAVIORAL PROCEDURES

A variety of more traditional procedures are used when treating depressed children. These procedures are used to help the child gain some control over his or her life and depressive symptoms. Behavioral procedures help the child gain distance from his or her depressive thoughts, which facilitates cognitive restructuring. They also serve as a means of altering the child's depressive thinking. Included in the present discussion are activity scheduling, social-skills training, assertiveness training, and relaxation training accompanied by positive imagery.

Activity Scheduling

Depressed children lead a very sedentary life style. They are withdrawn and shy away from participation in enjoyable activities. Because of a variety of depressive symptoms including fatigue, hypochondriasis, and anhedonia, the depressed child often declines opportunities to participate in enjoyable activities. Rather, the child spends time alone, lost in thought. When involved in an activity, the activity is likely to be a passive and non-goal-directed one.

Activity scheduling is the purposeful planning of the child's involvement in pleasant or goal-directed activities. Once the plan has been developed, the child tries to carry out the plan. The scheduling is quite detailed and may involve scheduling what the child is going to do on an hourly basis. The degree of detail is related to the depth of the depression. The more severely depressed child requires more detailed planning, since he or she is so severely withdrawn and inactive. These youngsters need the additional structure to get them to follow through on the plans.

Implementation

The first step in the activity-scheduling process is to help the child recognize that there is a relationship between what the child does and how he or she feels. This rationale has been established previously during assessment or affective education and is reviewed if necessary when implementing this procedure. Most children, although not all children, can readily see that their mood is better when they are active.

The next step is to identify mood-enhancing pleasant activities for the child client and activities that need to be performed for the child to function adaptively (e.g., completion of homework or a science project). As noted in the related section on training in self-monitoring, the identification of mood-enhancing activities can be accomplished by reviewing the child's mood and activity graph. If the youngster is not self-monitoring mood and activities with pleasant events schedules, then the activities that have been identified as being reinforcing during the assessment phase of self-reinforcement can be targeted for enactment. Additional activities can be identified through a number of procedures.

Mood-enhancing activities can be identified through a less structured form of self-monitoring in which the child simply writes down the label of any activity that he or she enjoys. The child can be asked to go through a pleasant events schedule and check off the activities that he or she likes to do. Another assessment procedure is the interview. The child and his or her parents can be interviewed to identify activities that the child did frequently before the episode of depression.

It is equally important to identify activities that the child needs to complete to continue to function adaptively. There are many things the child needs to accomplish such as completing homework and long-term assignments. Similarly, the child may belong to a club or organization such as scouts. Within these organizations, the youngster may be responsible for completing tasks for the organization such as purchasing all of the food for a weekend camping trip. To identify such activities, it often is necessary to interview significant others in the child's life, including parents and teachers, in addition to the child him- or herself.

Failure to complete these tasks can confirm a negative sense of self. The child who feels worthless or useless can cite as evidence his or her failure to complete such meaningful activities when justifying these negative self-evaluations. Additionally, the child may expend a great deal of energy worrying about whether he or she will complete or fail the task.

After identifying the relevant activities, the child and therapist create an activity schedule for the interim days before the next session. A copy of a form that facilitates the scheduling process can be found in Appendix N. The child and therapist go through the schedule sheet on an hour-by-hour basis and schedule the child's activities. Both pleasant activities and the completion of subgoals of task assignments are worked into the schedule. After completion of the schedule, the therapist and child try to identify potential impediments to following the schedule. Once possible impediments are identified, the child and therapist use problem solving to develop plans to overcome the roadblocks if they should arise.

It is very difficult for a child to complete the schedule as it is laid out. Unforeseen problems arise that the child has no control over. Thus, it is of critical importance for the therapist to inform the child that things are bound to happen that would impede the youngster's ability to complete the schedule. The best that the child can expect is that he or she puts forth some effort to try to become more active and to use these activities to control his or her mood.

Finally, the youngster is instructed to self-monitor his or her enactment of the schedule. Problems following the schedule are noted and worked out later with the therapist. As the child follows the schedule, he or she records the degree of mastery or pleasure that is experienced.

Graded Task Assignment

There are a number of variants of the activity-scheduling procedure that are quite useful. As mentioned in the previous section, it often is necessary for the therapist to work with the child to identify tasks that he or she needs to complete. Beck and colleagues (1979) refer to such tasks as graded task assignments. Sometimes the therapist might want to concentrate on helping the child to schedule the completion of these tasks. Such a situation would arise when the child feels extreme pressure and as though he or she is in a bind.

In such instances, the first step is to define the task to be mastered. For example, the child may have to complete a science project. Once the task is identified, it is broken down into subgoals or steps that have to be mastered along the way to task completion. For example, choosing a topic, finding relevant information, reading it, outlining the paper, and writing it one paragraph at a time are all subgoals to completion of the science project. As the therapist and child identify subgoals, the therapist elicits the child's thoughts about his or her chances of being able to complete the step. The child might believe that he or she is incapable of completing the task.

As the child works toward task completion, the therapist assesses the youngster's self-evaluations about subgoal attainment. Since depressed children have a tendency to evaluate their performances negatively, it is necessary to process the child's progress with him or her so that accomplishments are not discounted. In addition, the therapist coaches the child to make internal attributions for his or her accomplishments toward goal attainment. Internal attributions are only encouraged when it is realistic to attribute responsibility to the self.

After the child accomplishes the first task, a second, more complex task is then chosen, and the process is repeated.

Cognitive Rehearsal

Sometimes depressed youngsters find it difficult to carry out an activity plan or a graded task assignment even though the youngster clearly possesses the prerequisite skills. Cognitive rehearsal can be used to facilitate task completion.

After identifying the task to be completed and brainstorming the development of a plan, the client is led through an imaginary trip to task completion. The child, following the therapist's guidance, images completing each step of the task. While imaging, the child strives to experience the positive affect associated with task completion. A coping model is used during imagery as the therapist includes possible impediments to successful task completion as well as ways to overcome these roadblocks. After the child has successfully completed the task in his or her mind, the therapist reviews the steps to task completion with the child and then instructs the child to self-monitor progress following the plan.

Social-Skills Training

There is some evidence that indicates that depressed children are less popular than their nondepressed peers (Vosk, Forehand, Parker, & Richard, 1982). Our research (Linn & Stark, 1990) indicates that this lack of popularity may result from a disturbance in social skills. This disturbance is comprised of a skills deficit, a disturbance in cognitions surrounding social situations, and greater attention to physiological arousal.

Depressed children are described by themselves as well as their teachers as exhibiting significantly more inappropriately assertive behavior and significantly less appropriate social behavior. When entering social situations, and during a social interaction, depressed children think significantly more negative thoughts. They expect to be rejected and to make fools of themselves. As a result of the negative expectations and other thoughts, the youngster experiences heightened emotional arousal. This arousal is interpreted as further evidence that something bad is going to happen, which leads to further negative thinking. It appears as though a treatment for the social problems of depressed children must include both skills-training and cognitive restructuring components.

Social-skills training has been part of treatment programs for depressed children. It appears to have been one of the primary components in the "role-play" treatment utilized by Butler et al. (1980) (see Chapter 2). In the author's first treatment study, social-skills training was part of the "behavioral problem-solving" treatment. In the authors' current treatment program, social-skills training is used with those depressed children who appear to have a social problem.

A review of the existing social-skills-training studies with socially withdrawn (e.g., Bornstein, Bellack, & Hersen, 1977), aggressive (Elder, Edelstein, & Narick, 1979), and rejected children (Bierman, Miller, & Stabb, 1987) suggests that the training is effective. However, modifications to these programs appear to be necessary for depressed children. Specifically, greater attention needs to be paid to the cognitions of the child and to the subtle behaviors that set the child apart from his or her peers.

The therapist can identify the targets of the skills training through a number of procedures. Perhaps the simplest, yet commonly overlooked procedure, is to observe the child's interactions with you and consider your own reactions to the youngster. The child's interactions with the therapist are a sample of his or her interpersonal behavior in general, although it may be somewhat different from how the child behaves with other children. Nonetheless, the observations provide the therapist with some information. It is equally important for the therapist to tune into his or her affective reaction to the youngster. It is highly likely that other people including other children will have a similar reaction to the youngster. If the therapist notices a negative reaction to the child, then this should serve as a cue to pay special attention to the child's behavior in order to identify what the child is doing to produce such a reaction in others. Systematic observation of the child interacting with other children is imperative. Close attention to sequences of behavior that culminate in negative reactions in others are of particular interest.

The goal of assessment is to identify the content of the social-skills training. Once that material is identified, education, modeling, rehearsal, coaching, and corrective feedback are used to help the child learn the appropriate behaviors. During the education phase, the child is made aware of what he is or is not doing that is leading to social difficulties. Advantages and disadvantages of this behavior are discussed. Additionally, other more socially appropriate behaviors are introduced. Concurrently, the child's thoughts surrounding the deficient behavior are assessed, and attention is paid to identifying thoughts that elicit and maintain the maladaptive social behavior.

The therapist models the desired behavior for the child and discusses situations where it is appropriate to enact it. Next, the therapist coaches (verbally guides) the child through enactment of the desired behavior. To make the training situation seem more realistic, the child and therapist role-play a relevant scenario. The first time through the role-play, the therapist plays the child and models the desired behavior. Subsequently the child and therapist switch roles. As the role-play progresses, the child's cognitions surrounding the situation and his or her behaviors are assessed. Where appropriate, the therapist models adaptive thoughts that are associated with the target behavior. Cognitive restructuring is used where appropriate. The role-playing continues, and the therapist provides corrective feedback until the child has mastered the desired behavior. Additional education and modeling may be necessary.

Relaxation and Positive Imagery Training

The author's research (e.g., Stark, Laurent, et al., 1990) indicates that the most common co-occurring pathology with depression is anxiety. Especially common is persistent, excessive worry. To help the depressed child cope with this chronic anxiety, relaxation training is taught as a coping skill. Once again, cognitive restructuring procedures are needed to alter the cognitions regarding threat that underlie the worry. Relaxation also is used as a means of helping the youngster overcome the anxiety associated with targeted social or assertive behavior. Some children are extremely reluctant to try out their new behavior for fear of failure or negative repercussions. In these cases, imaging a successful experience while in a relaxed state seems to help them actually attempt the desired behavior.

Relaxation has been used as a treatment procedure in its own right for depression among adolescents (Reynolds & Coates, 1986). However, it is just one component of the treatment program used to treat depressed children, and it is combined with positive, coping imagery.

There are a variety of relaxation procedures that can be used; however, we have chosen to use deep muscle relaxation. The standard procedure of progressively tensing and then relaxing various muscle groups is followed. Some modifications to the instructions are made for children and young adolescents. When preparing the child to begin, the child is given an overview of what is going to happen. After describing the procedure, the therapist emphasizes the fact that the child is in complete control of the situation and that the therapist is simply going to read a script that will guide the youngster's attention. This emphasis on the child being in control is necessitated by the fact that many children are intimidated by the procedure, and some perceive it to be "hypnosis" and are concerned that they will do or say something that they do not want to disclose. The child also is given control over making the decision to dim the lights in the room.

There is a certain degree of intimacy associated with the procedure, which leads some early adolescents to feel uncomfortable. Their discomfort is expressed through giggling and disruptions over the course of the exercise. Some of this disruptiveness can be assuaged by challenging their maturity before the exercise begins. It can be explained to them that the exercise is something that is more commonly used with adults but that you believe the youngsters are mature enough to handle it.

Ollendick and Cerney (1981) have offered a number of useful guidelines for developing an age-appropriate relaxation exercise. They suggest adjusting the length of the exercise to the age and attention span of the child. For younger children, fewer muscle groups would be covered during a session. With older children who presumably have a longer attention span, more muscle groups could be covered during the course of a session. To increase the child's involvement in the exercise, more creative instructions can be used. A good example are those used by Koeppen (1974). Older children can be encouraged to develop their own relaxation exercises. They may be asked to make their own tapes to practice listening to outside of therapy sessions.

Daily practice of relaxation at home is critical for the child to achieve the desired depth of relaxation as well as the necessary automaticity of relaxation induction. It usually takes a child four to six exercises before he or she experiences a truly relaxed state. Relaxation is a skill that improves over time. The child needs to be informed of this so that he or she does not expect to achieve a level of deep relaxation during the first session. Making a tape recording of one of the relaxation exercises is quite useful, since the child can be instructed to listen to it every day at home. As noted earlier, this speeds up the acquisition and mastery of this skill.

An adjunct to relaxation training is guided imagery. Guided imagery is a procedure involving the therapist, who verbalizes a scene that the child tries to image. The imagery scenario is used immediately after the child has achieved a state of relaxation. In other words, after the therapist has led the child through the relaxation inducement instructions, while the child is relaxed, the therapist asks the child to close his or her eyes and to try to imagine in as much detail as possible the scenes that the therapist is about to describe. Then the therapist leads the youngster through a therapeutically relevant scene.

The content of the scene can be anything. Generally a few guidelines are kept in mind when the scenes are developed. First, the scene needs to be individually tailored to the child. This means that the scene includes as much personally relevant information as possible so that it seems "real" for the child. The places, characters, and small details are drawn from, and describe, the child's life. Secondly, the degree to which the therapist provides the structure and details of the scenes varies according to the age of the child. With younger children, the therapist provides more structure and detail.

The scenario must be directly related to the present target of change. For example, if the child is being encouraged to use a new social skill while going along with his classmates on a school trip, then the therapist creates a scenario that involves the child successfully trying out the new skill. A final, although critical, guideline is that the scenario employs a coping model. During the scene, the child is faced with some possible hurdles, his or her self-doubts are voiced, and the child is shown overcoming the hurdles and successfully enacting the desired behavior. Finally, the interpersonal outcome is positive. An example of an imagery scenario can be found in Appendix O.

FAMILY INTERVENTION PROCEDURES

As noted in Chapter 2, depressed youngsters often come from disturbed families. The assessment and treatment of dysfunctional families are complex topics that have been covered in depth in recent volumes such as the one by Epstein, Schlesinger, and Dryden (1988). A comprehensive discussion of family therapy is beyond the scope of this text. The present discussion will focus on concerns that, although important across childhood disorders, may be especially relevant for depression when it occurs in children.

Assessment

The primary means of assessing what is happening in the family is to join the family and experience and observe what goes on. Of primary interest to the cognitive–behavioral family therapist are the following questions: What behavior is being exhibited, or what verbiage is being stated, that communicates a message to the child that leads to and maintains the child's depressogenic thinking? What thoughts underlie various maladaptive behaviors of the family members? Thus, the therapist is looking for messages to the child that he or she is in some way bad or deficient, that the world is hostile, and/or that the future is bleak. For example, a parent who rejects a child physically (e.g., resists a hug) or verbally (e.g., "I wish you had never been born") is sending the child a message that he or she is not lovable, which leads to the development and maintenance of a negative self-schema. A family where the parents are unpredictably punitive (e.g., an alcoholic family) and/or say things such as "This is a rotten world. I hate it!" may lead to the development of a negative world schema. A negative schema for the future could develop in a child who comes from a family where aversive things happen to the child regardless of what the child does and/or where the child hears such things as "This world is just getting more and more screwed up" or "You'll always be no good." It also is evident from these examples that there are multiple messages in each statement or action.

It is not the author's contention that a single occurrence of one of these things will lead to the development of a maladaptive schema. Rather, it is the repeated occurrence of such messages over the developmental years that leads to the development of schemas that direct the child's attention and way of deriving meaning from the world in a negative and distorted way. It is very possible that the child's core schemas about him- or herself and the world start forming during the attachment period and solidify over time through repeated learning experiences.

From the moment of birth forward, the child begins receiving messages about him- or herself and the world. As these messages are encoded and stored, cognitive structures form, and the cognitive content ("propositions"; Ingram & Kendall, 1986) within the structures begins to accumulate. In addition, the rules or operations that direct the flow of information begin forming. As the child's cognitive structures develop, they begin to guide the processing of incoming, new information. The child's attention is directed toward schema-consistent information, which further solidifies the existing schemas. Thus, the child becomes an active constructor of his or her own reality. The youngster begins to act on the world as perceived rather than the world as it really is. In the psychologically disturbed child, there is a chasm between the world as perceived and reality. In the case of depressed youths, there is a negative distortion that stems from the dysfunctional schemas (cognitive structures and propositions) that have developed through the child's experiences with the world. Since the family plays such a major and influential role in the child's experiential learning, it is the therapist's job to identify those behaviors and verbal statements that communicate information to the child that further develops and maintains the child's maladaptive thinking.

A variety of phenomena within the family should be observed when one is trying to develop a treatment plan. As noted above, the family's interactional behaviors and verbal communications are observed in an effort to identify those behaviors and verbalizations that maintain the child's depressogenic thinking. Concurrently, the child's own behavior is observed to discover the role that he or she unwittingly plays in the maladaptive interactions and verbal communications. For example, the child may enact aversive behavior that quite naturally elicits a response that can be interpreted as rejection.

When observing and interacting with the family, it is important to try to identify maladaptive rules that may be governing the family's interactions and communications. These rules may become internalized by the child, or they may be misinterpreted and internalized by the child. For example, a covert family rule might be that you do not express any emotion or mom will become very upset and punish you. The child may perceive this as a communication that feelings are bad, that he or she is bad for having such feelings, or that no one cares about his or her feelings. The rules that govern the family's behavior may have to be deduced from observing and interacting with the family.

From the literature reviewed in Chapter 2, it seems as though it would be important to be alert for conflict within the family. Does the conflict pervade all aspects of the family, or is it specific to an individual, a pair of individuals, or some other combination. Is the conflict between the marital partners? What triggers the conflict?

How frequently does it occur? What terminates the conflict? How severe are the conflicts? Does the conflict escalate to violence? What do other family members do while the conflict occurs? These and other questions should be answered.

Another very important consideration from the literature appears to be the activity level of the family. Does the family restrict its recreational activities, social interactions, religious activity, and involvement in intellectual or cultural activities? What does the family do for fun? Why do they not do more? What would be necessary for the family to become more active? What are the parent's attitudes toward recreation?

From the literature reviewed in Chapter 2, it appears as though it is important for the therapist to ascertain how the family is managed. The reader may remember that depressed children tended to describe their families as less democratic. The most basic questions are: Do the parents run the family, or has a child been given the responsibility? If the parents manage the family, how do they manage it? Are they autocratic, laissez-faire, or do they balance being in charge with giving the children some input into decisions that directly affect them? In a related vein, how do the parents manage the children's behavior? Do they use positive techniques, punitive procedures, or some balance between the two? If punitive procedures are used, are they psychologically damaging such as guilt or shame inducement?

A number of the structural characteristics of the family also would be evaluated. These characteristics are described in greater detail by Stark and Brookman (in press). The structural characteristics of interest include the subsystems, boundaries, alignment, and power within the family. Elsewhere (Stark & Brookman, in press), we have hypothesized that the families of depressed children would be characterized by a weak marital subsystem, diffuse parent–child boundaries (enmeshment), low levels of supportive alliance behaviors, stable and detouring coalitions, and that these patterns of interaction are inflexible.

Treatment Issues

As our treatment has evolved over the years, the family component has grown in importance, as has the amount of time spent working with the depressed child's family. As a result of the assessment conducted during the first few meetings, a treatment plan is formulated. This plan will evolve as more is learned and as procedures are found to be effective or ineffective. Dependent on the outcome of the assessment, the family may serve as a treatment agent or focal point of intervention.

In the case of the relatively healthy family, the parents will be taught skills for aiding in the treatment of their child. The parents may be asked to remind the child to complete his or her self-monitoring assignments or other homework. They may be asked to aid in the child's attempts to self-reinforce. The parents can provide the child with the resources he or she needs to deliver material and activity rewards. They also might be taught how to identify maladaptive thoughts in their child. Once they are capable of doing this, they can remind the child to use his or her cognitive restructuring procedures. If the child is having some difficulty using cognitive restructuring, then the parents could be taught to help the child. The parents also might be instructed to gently encourage their depressed child to become involved in family activities, school activities, athletics, or regular exercise. Emphasis is placed on using positive inducements. Furthermore, the parents might be instructed to help the child become more socially active or to be accepting of their child's attempts to be more assertive. If their child is working toward self-improvement, then the parents may be asked to help the child carry out his or her plan. Finally, the parents might be instructed to counter certain irrational beliefs the child holds through specific things they say or do. For example, the parents may be instructed to verbalize observations about the positive qualities of their child.

Another consideration that influences the direction of treatment is the mental health of the parents and other family members. It is not uncommon to find another seriously psychologically disturbed member of the family. It is especially problematic when it is one of the parents. In such instances, the parent's problems can undermine the child's and family's treatment. Thus, it is wise to refer the parent for therapy and to consult with the parent's therapist if consent to do so can be secured. In some instances, it becomes necessary to consult with the mental health professionals who work with the parent following hospitalization. This often involves consulting with another team of psychologists who are conducting family therapy in conjunction with the treatment of the parent.

In the case of the disturbed family, the dysfunctional interactions and communications identified through the assessment process become the target of change. Parents are only asked to aid in the treatment process in the areas where they can do so effectively and without increasing the probability of a destructive interaction.

A variety of procedures can be employed following an assessment period and some educating of the family. The education process involves both helping them to understand the cognitive–behavioral perspective and how it applies to their family and to understand how to become active observers of their own interactions. This observation process helps them to become aware of the existence, parameters, and magnitude of dysfunctional interactions. They also are taught to try to identify the underlying messages that they are communicating to one another. The therapist is very active during this time, educating, pointing out examples of dysfunctional interactions, and modeling how to recognize the content of the messages being communicated and the thoughts of the recipient of the message.

The therapist may use directives to change the behavior of family members. The new behavior commonly is tried out within the session where the therapist can coach, model, and provide feedback. In addition, it provides the family with a forum where the impact of the new behavior can be discussed. Furthermore, reasons why the behavior would not be enacted can be identified, and plans for overcoming these impediments can be developed.

Problem-solving skills are taught to the family in an analogous manner to the way in which the child is taught problem solving. During the sessions, family members and the therapist identify problems that need to be resolved. The therapist models and coaches the family members through the seven steps of the problem-solving sequence. The objective of the training is to get the family members to use problem solving independently to prevent and resolve conflicts and to be able to deal better with the many unexpected events that one faces.

As therapy progresses and maladaptive family rules are discovered, they are brought to the family's attention. They are presented as hypotheses to be tested rather than as facts. The family is asked to try on the rule as a means of validating or invalidating it. If the therapist's deductions are accurate and such a rule exists, then the family and therapist work toward modifying it. This commonly involves using the cognitive-restructuring procedures described in Chapter 4. These procedures may be used with a single family member who is the harbinger of the rule, or they may be used with the entire family in an attempt to help them give it up. In addition, since the rule may have served some functional utility, it may be necessary to have the family use problem solving to develop a more adaptive rule.

Helping the family recognize the parameters of the conflict (who is involved; what precedes and maintains it) is a first step toward reducing it. Depending on the specifics of the conflict, the therapist may want to teach the family members first to recognize early signs that a conflict is developing and then to use those signs as cues to remain calm, use problem solving to develop a plan, and express oneself assertively. They also may have to be taught how to negotiate.

Similar to the treatment of the inactive depressed child, activity scheduling can be used to increase the activity level of the inactive family. This should be accomplished in a fashion that involves input from all members and in a way that recognizes the family's financial and practical constraints. Children commonly want to do things like go to "Great America" theme park or to "Sea World." Although these are a good deal of fun and can be entertaining for everyone, they also are very expensive adventures. The therapist does not want to encourage actions that will lead to financial pressures and greater stress. The parents, in contrast, often come up with very sendentary suggestions (rent a video), or they feel hopeless because of financial constraints. Thus, the therapist needs to be aware of low-cost/no-cost family entertainment. There actually are quite a few things than can be done, including playing cards, board games, catch, tennis, basketball, swimming, going for a walk, going to a park, museum, or library. School activities also are a very good resource. The family may just need to be educated about what is available in their own home and community.

Often it is necessary to elicit the thoughts of various family members surrounding engagement in pleasant activities. A parent may hold some irrational beliefs about enjoying oneself. Another very important consideration is the degree of conflict in the family. Will directing the family to do something together increase the probability of conflict? If so, then activity scheduling should be delayed until the family members have acquired skills for handling conflicts.

If the time is right for directing the family to engage in pleasant activities, and the family can choose some that they can all agree on (this is a good opportunity to teach negotiation skills), then the therapist works with the family to plan the activities (e.g., what, when, and where). In addition, the therapist probes the family to identify potential impediments to carrying out the plan. Problem solving is used to develop possible solutions for these potential impediments.

In the case of the family that is out of control or overly punitive, the parents can be taught basic behavior-management skills. Emphasis is placed on managing the children's behavior through positive procedures. In addition, parents are instructed to try the least aversive punishment procedures possible when it is necessary to use punishment. Furthermore, consistency, carry through, and making the consequence fit the behavior are some of the principles that are emphasized with the parents. The sessions often provide the therapist with an ideal opportunity to model the implementation of various behavior-management techniques. In addition, the parent can be coached through the process during the sessions.

When the parents do not allow their children any say in the decision-making process, an attempt is made to change this so that the parents remain in charge but the children are given the opportunity to have some input. The goal is to find a balance between the parents being in charge and the children feeling as though they have a reasonable amount of say in decisions that affect them. In some instances, it is necessary to do some cognitive restructuring with the parents in order for them to be able to give up some control. Likewise, a child may be instructed to keep track of how many times his or her parents involve him or her in decisions.

In order to change dysfunctional structural characteristics, a variety of procedures can be used, including support, education, coaching, modeling, and corrective feedback. In addition, parent training in behavior-management procedures may be used to decrease the permeability of the boundaries between the parents and children. A secondary effect may be the strengthening of the parental coalition. Homework assignments that produce a change in behavior or the education of the family can be given.

ESTABLISHING A THERAPEUTICALLY PRODUCTIVE SCHOOL ENVIRONMENT

Over the years of working with depressed children in the schools, it has become acutely apparent that the school psychologist's impact as a therapist is greatly enhanced or impeded by support or lack thereof from the child's teachers and administrators. If school personnel cooperate and participate, treatment is more effective. If the teachers do not cooperate, then the treatment program often is undermined. What can be done to enlist the support and cooperation of the child's teachers as well as other school personnel? What are areas where their support is needed?

The treatment program that has been described is a time-consuming program that removes the child from the classroom for 1½ to 2 hours per week. Some teachers object to this because they believe that it detracts from the child's academic advancement. Furthermore, it can create more work for the teacher as he or she has to make special arrangements for the child to get any assignments or materials that the youngster has missed. Additionally, the child's coming and going at odd times can create a minor disturbance for the class. In some ways, the child's treatment also threatens the teacher's sense of effectiveness, since teachers often feel as though they should be able to meet all of their students' needs.

When such beliefs exist, the teacher's ensuing behavior can undermine treatment. For example, we have experienced teachers who have mandated that the child can only leave the classroom for one 20-minute period or that the child can only leave during certain nonacademic classes or that the child can only be removed from free times such as recess, lunch, or P.E. In one instance, a child's teacher refused to give a child the assignments that he missed while in the therapist's office. Perhaps the worst incident was a teacher who gave a fourth-grade girl a failing grade for the 6-week period because she had missed too much time because of her participation in treatment.

We have found that steps can be taken to avoid such unfortunate incidents. First, it is critical to have support for the treatment services at the top level of administration. In our most productive school district, the superintendent has given us his complete support and has communicated this in writing to his school principals. In turn, the school principals have communicated their support for treatment to their staff through memos and verbally during faculty meetings. This support was achieved through pointing out the humanitarian and fiscal value of treatment. More expensive and long-lasting treatment can be avoided in the long run by teaching the children coping skills. In addition to the principals' general support for the children's involvement in treatment, the principals have advocated this attitude: The child is not learning as much as he or she could now because of the emotional problem, and he or she never will live up to his or her potential without treatment. Thus, class time lost to treatment now will be more than made up for in the long run.

We have made a point of consulting with each child's teacher(s). They are involved in the assessment process; they are engaged in the process; of individualizing the treatment program; and they are challenged to help develop means of translating the treatment procedures for classroom use with the child. Some teachers have been very creative and effective in this regard. Furthermore, the teacher may be consulted with to determine whether there are any ways the workload could be temporarily reduced for the child.

An overlooked advantage of this consultation is the visibility it provides the psychologist. The teacher may be meeting the psychologist for the first time. It helps teachers see that the psychologist provides a useful service and that he or she is not simply spending time fiddling around in the office.

More direct attempts to increase the psychologist's visibility have been made. The school psychologists have done in-services and workshops for the teachers. Evening parent presentations have been conducted in which the teachers may be participants.

Finally, perhaps the best promotional tool is treatment success. As the teachers recognize the change in a child, they tell other teachers and cooperation spreads.

SUMMARY

In the previous two chapters a comprehensive treatment program for depressed children was described. The program combines behavioral, self-control, and cognitive procedures that are used with the child with family therapy procedures. The behavioral and self-control procedures are used to help the depressed child learn how to cope with depressive symptoms, to gain some objectivity toward his or her thoughts, and to produce cognitive change. Cognitive procedures are used to change the automatic thoughts, schemas, and core schemas that underlie the depressive symptoms and maladaptive behavior patterns. Family therapy procedures are used to change the interactions and verbal communications within the family that lead to, and maintain, the child's maladaptive behaviors and cognitions.

The techniques that are chosen to comprise the treatment program vary across children. The procedures are chosen to meet the individual child's needs based on the results of a comprehensive cognitive–behavioral assessment of the child and his or her environment. Thus, the child's treatment program is individually tailored to meet the child's psychosocial needs. The procedures serve as a vehicle for producing three primary objectives. The first is changing the way that the child derives meaning from his/her world. To this end, change at the level of core cognitive structures is sought. The second primary objective is to teach the child a set of cognitive and behavioral skills that he or she can use on his or her own to control depressive symptomatology. The third objective is to alter the events in the child's environment that are leading to and maintaining the child's depressogenic thinking and behaviors.

Although the techniques seem to be relatively simple and straightforward to implement, it takes quite a bit of skill and practice to be able successfully and skillfully to choose the combination of procedures needed to produce the desired change. Clients commonly report some symptom improvement during the sessions. In fact, the child may exhibit marked improvement as a result of cognitive restructuring that is directed toward schematic change. However, it is important to note that this symptom relief probably will be temporary. It takes repeated learning experiences, not just one eloquent use of a cognitive restructuring procedure, to produce lasting change. Furthermore, the treatment is not complete until the child has learned to apply the procedures independently on a moment-by-moment basis as needed. It also is important to note that long-term change may only be possible following an alteration in the child's environment. This includes a change in family communications, interactions, and maladaptive rules. In the case of the depressed child who is having difficulty in school, the child's educational program may have to be altered to reflect the child's diminished intellectual ability.

Experience suggests that the vast majority of depressed youths progress through school without being identified or receiving any treatment. It is hoped that this book will serve as some impetus for reversing this unfortunate situation. There is some evidence to suggest that the prevalence of depression is on the increase for a variety of social reasons. With these trends likely to continue or worsen, and with the schools being expected to play a greater role in the psychological care of our youths, it is going to be important for school psychologists to become more proficient at identifying and helping disturbed youths. It is hoped that this book, as a part of the larger School Practitioner's Series, will aid school psychologists in this endeavor.

Appendices

APPENDIX A
Transcription of an Interview with a Moderately Depressed Middle-School Student

K-SADS INTERVIEW

Gender: Female
Chronological age: 14–3
Grade: 7

Interviewer: Are there any kinds of troubles, worries, problems, or things that you can tell me are going on with you?

Child: Well, um, my friends . . . we've been having problems.

I: You're having problems with your friends?

C: I'm getting into fights with them a lot.

I: What kind of fights?

C: You know, just arguments and then not talking to each other.

I: I see. Is this something that just started recently, or is this something that has been a problem for a long time?

C: It started a little while ago.

I: How are you doing in school?

C: Not too well.

I: Has that always been a problem?

C: No.

I: How long has that been a problem?

C: Since this school year began.

I: How do you get along with your parents?

C: Fine.

I: O.K., so you have some problems with your friends and your school work. Are those your main worries, or are there other kinds of things that bother you?

C: Well, my parents get upset when I don't make good grades.

I: What do your parents do when you make poor grades?

C: They ground me until I get a good report card.

I: How were your grades this last report card?

C: They were C's and D's.

I: Is that good enough for them?

C: Well, as long as I don't have low C's.

I: Do you like school, or how do you feel about school?

C: I don't like the classes.

I: Do you get along with the teachers?

C: Yes.

I: Do you think of yourself as a happy person or a sad person? How do you see yourself?

C: Sometimes happy and sometimes sad.

I: Up and down?

C: Yes.

I: In the last 7 days have you been sad or down?

C: No.

I: During the past year have you been feeling sad or depressed?

C: Yes.

I: What does it feel like when you feel depressed?

C: Like when someone hurts your feelings.

I: And you feel real down? Or like if you did real crummy and your parents got on to you and you felt real yucky and you didn't want to be around people and you kind of hung out in your room or something?

C: That's what I've been doing for the last year. I just come home and go up into my room and sit around and read.

I: You don't feel like you have a whole lot of energy?

C: Uh huh.

I: Was it like that way last year?

C: No.

I: So it's been during this past school year you began feeling that way?

C: Uh huh.

I: Did you feel that way during the summer?

C: Just sat around.

I: You were just kind of bored?

C: Yes.

I: But last year you didn't feel that way?

C: Yes.

I: Do you have any idea why you started to feel that way this past year?

C: No. My mom says it's cause I'm getting older.

I: All right, so this whole past year it sounds like you have been feeling the same. Kind of blah. Every day you feel that way?

C: Ya.

I: O.K, so most days do you feel kind of down or blah? Like more than half the day, or pretty much all the time?

C: Not all the time.

I: About half the time?

C: Ya.

I: This kind of down and blah feeling you have, is it the same kind of feeling you get when someone moves away? Or like when your friend moves away? Is it a lonely kind of feeling, or is it different?

C: Different.

I: A lot different, or sort of?

C: Some different.

I: How is it different? Like have you ever had a pet die or something like that where you felt real bad?

C: Two weeks ago.

I: Oh really? O.K., but this general blah feeling you have . . . is it kind of different from how you felt when you felt bad about your pet?

C: I just feel real draggy.

I: Just feel draggy?

C: Yes.

I: Do you always know why you feel that way?

C: No.

I: Do you sometimes know why, or do you never know why?

C: *(Nods to "sometimes.")*

I: You sometimes know why?

C: *(Nods.)*

I: If somebody tries to cheer you up, can they do it?

C: *(Nods.)*

I: All the way or just some of the way?

C: Sometimes.

I: Sometimes they can cheer you up all the way?

C: *(Nods.)* . . . I haven't been eating anything lately.

I: Were you feeling draggy like that this past week?

C: Ya?

I: Since when did you stop feeling like eating?

C: This year. I've been losing weight and not eating.

I: You're not hungry?

C: No.

I: Are you trying to lose weight or are you just not hungry?

C: Just not hungry.

I: Do your parents try to get you to eat?

C: My mom said she would ground me if I didn't eat. I'm just not eating.

I: Uh huh. O.K. . . . Do you feel draggy more in the evening, morning, or in the afternoon, or is it just the same?

C: Afternoon.

I: Afternoon? A lot worse than in the mornings or just some worse?

C: Some *(almost a whisper)*.

C: I haven't been getting much sleep either.

I: You have a hard time sleeping? Going to sleep, or when you wake up, or what?

C: Just restless.

I: O.K. Now let's talk about getting mad. Do you get mad much?

C: Ya.

I: What kinds of things do you get mad about?

C: When I don't get my way.

I: This past week, that is this past 7 days, have you gotten mad during that time?

C: *(Nods.)*

I: Tell me about it.

C: It was about my friend. O.K. We were best friends, and she went to this city over spring break, and she did a lot of things that I haven't done. I didn't eat at all that week. She. . . .

I: What did she do?

C: My cousin gave her a skateboard, and she was going on talking all about that, making me feel bad. Like she hasn't given me one. And I got mad at her. She thinks that she is Miss Universe or something. . . . Well, we're friends now but cause Ms. P had us talk it out Monday, and . . . she's having family problems now.

I: So that's been kind of getting at you.

C: *(Nods.)*

I: Do you feel worse since you have been having problems than you did before?

C: No.

I: No? Doesn't sound like you have really made up.

C: We're really tired of each other. We have been with each other for a year, and we always spend every day together. We're just tired of each other.

I: Do you fight much with your older sister?

C: *(Nods.)*

I: Lots or some?

C: It hasn't been too bad.

I: This past 7 days have you felt mad pretty much?

C: No.

I: No? You haven't gotten mad at all?

C: No not recently.

I: Like when you all talked with Ms. P on Monday, were you mad at her then?

C: We didn't talk to her; we were talking by ourselves.

I: How long had you been mad at her?

C: A long time. . . . she just didn't know it.

I: Did you feel mad like every day or not all the time?

C: Sometimes. I just didn't really care.

I: Well, do you think during the past 7 days you felt mad as much as 3 times during the 7-day period?

C: *(Nods "no.")*

I: You weren't mad that much?

C: Saturday was when I was really upset.

I: How about being mad about other things?

C: *(Nods "no.")*

I: No? How about during this last 12 months, between now and last March? Has there been a time when you got mad a real lot?

C: My dad and I got in an argument.

I: Was it something you were mad about for just a short while or for a long time?

C: A couple of days.

I: Do you ever get so mad that you want to hurt somebody or break things?

C: Uh huh.

I: And you shout and lose your temper?

C: Sometimes *(low voice)*.

I: About how often do you think that happens?

C: Not very often.

I: When you are mad, do you always know why?

C: Most of the time. Sometimes I just start crying for no reason.

I: Uh huh. Has that happened this last week?

C: A couple of weeks ago.

I: Can someone or something cheer you up when you are mad and make you stop being mad?

C: They can make me forget about it for a little while.

I: For how long? . . . Like for an hour or longer than that?

C: Longer than that.

I: Do you get mad more in the morning or in the afternoon or evening?

C: Afternoon *(whispers)*.

I: A lot more in the afternoon or just some more?

C: Some more *(whispers)*.

I: Do you know what it means to feel guilty?

C: I don't know.

I: O.K. Like if you did something wrong and you think it's your fault. And maybe you even tell the person you're sorry, but you still keep feeling bad about it. Does that happen to you much? Do you ever feel like things are your fault even when you didn't do it?

C: *(Nods "no.")*

I: Are you pretty satisfied with what your personality is like? . . . How you act?

C: Sometimes.

I: Sometimes you get down on yourself about it?

C: *(Nods "yes.")*

I: O.K. Are you satisfied with the way you look?

C: *(Nods "no.")*

I: So it sounds like you kind of feel down about yourself in some ways. Would you say real down or just kind of down?

C: Kind of down.

I: Do you ever feel like you hate yourself and are just worthless?

C: *(Nods "yes.")*

I: Have you felt that way this last week, in the last 7 days, like you weren't worth anything?

C: Ya.

I: During the past year have there been times when you felt worthless?

C: When people laugh at me and make fun of me.

I: And why do people do that?

C: People at my church do all the time cause I'm in junior high. I'm the only junior high person in there, and the rest of them are high schoolers and they just laugh at me.

I: What church do you go to?

C: _____ Church.

[break]

I: O.K., we were talking about feeling down on yourself. You said you would like to change how smart you are, how you look, and what your personality is like. You'd like to change these things?

C: I guess my personality is O.K.

I: Do you ever feel like nobody cares about you?

C: *(Nods.)*

I: Have you felt that way this past week, like no one cared?

C: Last night.

I: Why? Was there anything that made you feel that way?

C: My mom . . . she told my sister that she could do what ever she wanted, and she made me clean the kitchen.

I: So you got mad and felt that nobody cared. Were there any other times this past week when you felt that no one cared?

C: Sunday, um . . . I am the only junior high person and they wouldn't let me go with them. The high school group.

I: Is your church kind of small?

C: Uh huh.

I: Do you think that you are real concerned about people not caring or just kind of every once in a while?

C: Kind of.

I: Do you think things will get better? Do you feel like things in the future will be pretty much positive and good things will happen, or do you think things will be bad?

C: You mean as in jobs or something?

I: Any parts of your life, like doing better in school or getting along better with your friends. Do you think better things will happen?

C: I don't know about school.

I: How about your friends?

C: Probably.

I: Do you think that life has been harder for you than for your friends?

C: No.

I: Do you have aches and pains much like headaches, stomachaches . . . not like when you have the flu or something?

C: Headaches.

I: Like how many headaches have you had in the last 7 days?

C: Three.

I: How about this last year. Is that pretty much how it is each week, about three headaches . . . a little less or a little more?

C: Sometimes. . . . Sometimes less and sometimes more. This past week I've been having them a lot. I get migraine headaches too.

I: Do you have to go to bed?

C: Uh huh.

I: Do you get sick to your stomach?

C: *(Nods "yes.")*

I: What do you take?

C: Just Nuprin. After a while it goes away.

I: About how often do you get those?

C: I haven't had one in a while, but they've been real bad.

I: Do you ever feel like you're getting some kind of disease?

C: *(Nods "no.")*

I: Are you bored much?

C: Uh huh.

I: Like more than you used to be when you were younger? Are you bored with things that you should enjoy?

C: I usually have a good time, but when I sit at home and watch TV. I don't like to watch TV.

I: That can get boring, doing that. Do you get tired a lot?

C: *(Nods "yes.")*

I: Do you think a lot more than most kids your age? Do you have to rest when you get home from school?

C: Oh ya.

I: Do you feel tired almost all the time or just sometimes?

C: A lot of the time.

I: And it has been this way this last week?

C: Uh huh.

I: And this last year?

C: Uh huh.

I: Do you have problems paying attention, like in class . . . even when you want to pay attention do you have a hard time?

C: *(Nods "yes.")*

I: Does it get in the way of your doing O.K. in school?

C: Uh huh.

I: Do you forget things a lot?

C: *(Nods "yes.")*

I: Is it a real bad problem or just a problem?

C: Just a problem. That's why I'm having a problem in school, cause I might forget to bring a certain book home or something.

I: Is it stuff that you study for?

C: Uh huh.

I: Do you have problems sitting still?

C: Sometimes.

I: But it's not a real big problem for you?

C: *(Nods "no.")*

I: Do you have problems getting going, like once you sit still you'd just as soon not move? Like do your arms and legs feel heavy? Is that a problem for you?

C: Sometimes.

I: When feeling draggy and down do you notice that you talk slower or quieter than other times, or do you pretty much talk the same?

C: The same.

I: Do you like to be around other people or by yourself or both? When you go shut yourself up in your room when you get home from school, would you rather be by yourself then?

[long pause]

I: Are you shutting yourself up away from your family, or what are you doing?

C: I want to be someplace where there's not a lot of people.

I: O.K., but some?

C: Uh huh.

I: Are you satisfied with your friends? It sounds like you've got some problems with them? Do you wish you had different friends?

C: Sometimes . . . when we're in a fight or something.

I: But you would generally rather spend time with your friends than by yourself?

C: Uh huh.

I: O.K. You said you had trouble sleeping. Do you have trouble falling asleep at night?

C: No . . . just. . . .

I: Can't stay asleep?

C: Ya . . . and then after . . . um . . . I've been having trouble I'll wake up and I won't be able to get up and I'll hit my alarm four times.

I: O.K. Do you wake up in the middle of the night sometimes and can't go back to sleep? Did you do that this past week?

C: Uh huh.

I: How many times?

C: A lot.

I: Like every night?

C: Uh huh.

I: And once you wake up, how long do you stay awake?

C: About 20 minutes.

I: Do you ever wake up too early in the morning?

C: No.

I: You just sleep restlessly like you don't feel like you slept when you wake up?

C: Uh huh.

I: Real bad or just some?

C: Bad.

I: And you're sleepy during the day?

C: Uh huh. And, see, if I go to bed early I can't go to sleep.

I: On the weekends do you sleep for hours and hours and can't get up?

C: *(Nods "no.")*

I: All right, and you don't want to eat. Is that right?

C: Uh huh.

I: Less than you did . . . say last year?

C: *(Nods "no.")*

I: When did you start not wanting to eat?

C: A couple of months ago I just. . . .

I: So it hasn't been going on this whole last year, just the last couple of months.

C: *(Nods "yes.")*

I: When was it the worst?

C: Just this past few months.

I: And you've lost weight?

C: *(Nods "yes.")*

I: And you're not trying to diet; you just don't want to eat?

C: *(Nods "yes.")*

I: Would you say that you rarely feel hungry?

C: I'm hungry, but I just don't want to eat. I feel like I'm going to throw up or something when I think of food.

I: Do you think that you are fat?

C: *(Nods "yes.")*

I: Do you know you're not fat but just think that you might be fat? Or do you think that you really are fat?

C: I think I am.

I: So you feel like you are going to barf if you eat? Is it the food? You don't like the food, you don't like the thought of eating, or what?

C: I don't like to think of eating.

I: There's no certain things like candy bars you'd like to eat anyway?

C: I like to drink water . . . that's what I've been craving a lot.

I: But you're not just trying to lose weight? It just grosses you out to think of eating?

C: *(Nods "yes.")*

I: You say you feel hungry but you don't want to eat.

C: Uh huh.

I: How much weight do you think you've lost?

C: At least 7 or 8 pounds.

I: Your clothes fit differently and everything?

C: *(Nods "yes.")* A couple months ago during Christmas I was wearing . . . no . . . like in October I was wearing a 12 but now I'm wearing like a 6.

I: And this worries your parents some?

C: They just think it's weird.
I: So this last week do you feel like you've lost a little weight too?
C: Uh huh. I weighed myself Monday and I weighed 117 and then I weighed myself Sunday at 115.
I: So, do you weigh yourself pretty often?
C: Uh huh. Almost every day. See, everyone in my house is on a diet except me.
I: Is everyone a little overweight?
C: My sister and my dad are.
I: Kids who are having a hard time sometimes think about hurting themselves or killing themselves. Do you ever think about that kind of stuff?
C: *(Near whisper.)* Uh huh.
I: What did you do?
C: I ate a bunch of pills.
I: What kind of pills?
C: Tylenol.
I: When did you do that?
C: A couple of weeks ago when my dad and I had a really bad fight.
I: How many pills did you eat?
C: I'm not sure. Probably a dozen or so.
I: Did you stop eating them, or did you run out of them?
C: The bottle was empty.
I: Was anyone else at home when you did this?
C: Yes, my dad and sister.
I: Were they close by, like in the next room?
C: I guess so.
I: Did you really want to kill yourself, or did you just want to scare your dad?
C: I wanted to kill myself.
I: What ended up happening?
C: I got sick and threw them up. I told my dad it was something that I ate at school.
I: Have there been any other times this year that you tried to hurt yourself?
C: No.
I: Did you think about or try to kill yourself over the past 7 days?
C: No.
I: Have there been any times when you tried hurting yourself but not killing yourself? Like just cutting yourself, or burning yourself?
C: No.

APPENDIX B
Symptom Checklist

Please read each statement carefully. If the statement is true about how you felt over the last week, circle the number of that statement. If the statement is not true about you over the last week, then just read it and go on to the next statement.

1. I felt sad, or down, or unhappy, or like crying.
2. I was angry.
3. I felt guilty.
4. I felt like no one loved me.
5. I didn't like myself.
6. I felt like life was harder on me than on other people.
7. I had aches and pains.
8. I worried about my health.
9. I was tired.
10. I had trouble concentrating.
11. I couldn't sit still.
12. I felt like I was moving in slow motion.
13. I wanted to be by myself.
14. Nothing seemed fun.
15. I had trouble sleeping.
16. I slept longer than usual.
17. I didn't feel like eating.
18. I ate more than usual.
19. I tried to hurt myself.
20. I thought about hurting myself.

APPENDIX C
Goals and Subgoals for
Each of 21 Sessions

SESSION 1

Objective 1: *Introduction of therapists and participants*
   A. Acknowledge appreciation for the kids' participation.
   B. Set meeting days and times.
   C. Address confidentiality issue.
   D. Facilitate participant introductions.

Objective 2: *Begin building group cohesion*
   Activity 1: Getting to know you.
   Where you live.
   What you enjoy doing.
   What things you are good at.

Objective 3: *Give the participants a chance to discuss the parent interviews*
   Facilitate a discussion of the parent interviews.

Objective 4: *Identify the participants' specific concerns and perceptions of why they are in the group*
   A. Question each participant on why he or she is there.
   B. State reasons for attendance and objectives of treatment.
   C. Have participants write goals for themselves to achieve in the group.

SESSION 2

Objective 1: *Introduction to participants' agendas*

Objective 2: *Build group cohesion*
   Emotion vocabulary exercise.

Objective 3: *Introduction to the rationale: The relationship between behavior and mood*
   A. Summary of emotion vocabulary activity.
   B. Introduce cartoon sequence to portray the connection between mood and behavior (use real-life examples whenever possible).

Practice
   Recognize when you are sad, angry, or happy and write down what was happening, and what you were doing and thinking about (see Appendix D).

SESSION 3

Set Agenda

Review Practice
  A. Go over homework assignment, recognize feelings and thoughts.
  B. Have group members share their assignments.

Objective 1: *Review and extend the participants' understanding of the mood-behavior relationship*
  A. Tell Nicki's story.
  B. Relate the story to the mood–behavior relationship.

Objective 2: *Introduction to self-reinforcement*
  A. Rewards.
  B. Punishment.

Objective 3: *Introduction to self-consequation*
  Giving yourself rewards.

Objective 4: *Generate a list of potential rewards*
  A. Help participants recognize three major ways of rewarding themselves.
    • Give themselves something tangible.
    • Let themselves do something fun.
    • Think about something positive.
  B. Have participants generate a list of rewards for themselves.

Practice
  Reward yourself at least once, preferably more, and write it down. Note how it feels to reward yourself.

SESSION 4

Set Agenda

Review Practice
  Discuss the self-reward assignment.

Objective 1: *Emphasize the mood/reward relationship*
  A. Sad kids don't reward themselves as much, so don't forget to reward yourself.

Objective 2: *Introduce the idea of contingent administration of rewards*
  A. Using rewards as motivation.
  B. Finish the job before rewarding yourself.

Objective 3: *Generate additional rewards and introduce the idea that they vary in reward value*
  A. Use participants' own list of rewards for discussion and examples.
  B. Rank rewards: big, small, and medium.

    C. Make the connection between the size of the job/task and the rank of the reward (i.e., big job gets big rewards, etc.).

    D. Brainstorm examples of jobs and rewards for school and home.

Practice

Make note on your reminder sheet of any rewards you give yourself between our meetings.

SESSION 5

Set Agenda

Review Practice

    A. Go over any tasks completed and rewards given.

Objective 1: *Introduction to self-monitoring*

    A. Use cartoons to introduce the relationship between:

- Negative thoughts about self and feelings.
- Positive thoughts about self and feelings.
- Negative thoughts about the future and feelings.
- Only paying attention to the negative things that happen and feelings.

Objective 2: *Preparation for completing diary*

    A. Use 3 × 5 cards to represent each thought, event, or activity.

- Have participants use the cards to fill out their diaries.
- Have participants rate themselves as if the events had occurred.

    B. Remind participants to fill out their diary three times a day.

- Rate overall mood at end of day.
- Remember to bring booklet to the meeting.
- Reward yourself for keeping up with the diary.
- Generate list of rewards.
- Sign contract on agreement concerning the diaries.

Practice

Complete your diaries and pay close attention to your feelings.

SESSION 6

Set Agenda

Review Practice

    A. Review the diaries.

    B. Review the procedure concerning the diaries.

    C. Use cartoon sequence (Figure 3.4) as a reminder to fill out diaries.

    D. Remember to collect their completed diaries.

Objective 1: *Make the mood, behavior, thought, event relationship more concrete*

Explain the process for graphing the mood, behavior, thought, and event relationship using one member's diary.

Objective 2: *Overcoming depression through increasing pleasant activities*
   A. Use cartoon sequence to portray how what happens to you, what you do and think affects the way you feel.
   B. Have participants figure out their average number of positive events and thoughts.
   C. Set a goal for increasing pleasant events.
   D. Sign a contract stating each participants' commitment to achieving his or her goals.
   E. Have kids help each other figure out what they like to do.

Practice
   Remind participants to fill out their diaries.

SESSION 7

Set Agenda

Review Practice
   A. Go over participants' diaries.
   B. Figure average number of good things and thoughts since last meeting.
   C. Process any progress, or lack of, toward obtaining goal.

Objective 1: *Promote further increase in pleasant events (activities, events, and thoughts) levels*
   A. Set another goal toward increasing pleasant events.
   B. Remind the participants to enlist parental help and support.

Objective 2: *Begin teaching relaxation as a coping skill (deep muscle and imagined)*
   A. Introduce and give rationale.
   B. Go through relaxation exercise.
   C. Begin imagery exercise.
   D. Process the participants' relaxation and imagery experience.
   E. Cartoon sequence.

Practice
   A. Continue filling out diaries.
   B. Work on relaxing and using imagery.

SESSION 8

Set Agenda

Review Practice
   A. Review participants' diaries.

   B. Complete participants' graphs.
   C. Review participants' use of relaxation.
   D. Collect completed diaries.

Objective 1: *Help the participants to gain greater control over their environment through assertiveness training*
   A. Introduce this topic by distinguishing among aggressive, passive, and assertive behavior.
   B. Use cartoon sequence to illuminate.
   C. Have participants pick someone to approach assertively.
   D. Role-play assertive behavior with this person.

Objective 2: *Provide practice in relaxation if time permits*
Lead participants through deep muscle relaxation and imagery.

Practice
   A. Continue to fill out diaries.
   B. Approach the person you chose to do something assertive with.
   C. Remind participants to use relaxation skills.
   D. Therapists fill out assertiveness activity sheet.

SESSION 9

Set Agenda

Review Practice
   A. Go over the diaries.
   B. Fill in diary graphs.
   C. Remember to collect the completed diaries.

Review the Participants' Attempts at Assertiveness
Discuss how it went for each participant.

Objective 1: *Extend assertiveness skills to giving compliments*
Explain and emphasize assertiveness in regard to complimenting others.

Objective 2: *Role-play giving compliments to family and friends*
   A. Therapists use their own experiences as examples to begin role play.
   B. Have group members role-play giving compliments to the people they have chosen to compliment.

Objective 3: *Practice relaxation*

Objective 4: *Complete an easy, self-esteem enhancing exercise*
   A. Have each participant think of two things they like about themselves and tell the group.
   B. Have each participant think of three things they like about each of the other group members and take turns sharing with each group member.

Practice
   A. Complete diaries.

B. Remind participants to give compliments.

C. Practice relaxation.

D. Therapists fill out sheet on participants' compliments.

SESSION 10

Set Agenda

Review Practice

A. Therapists review diaries before the session to prepare for discussing trends.

B. Fill out diary graphs.

C. Collect participants' diaries.

D. Review participants' attempts to tell family members what they like about them

Objective 1: *Assertiveness training (telling people that they are doing something you don't like)*

A. Explain rationale for assertive behavior when people are doing something you don't like.

B. Introduce the three foci of the assertive statement:

• What the person is doing that you do not like.

• How it makes you feel.

• What you would like them to do instead.

Objective 2: *Practice relaxation*

Do a short relaxation and then image being assertive.

Practice

A. Continue to complete the diaries.

B. Ask someone, in an assertive manner, to stop doing something you don't like.

C. Therapists fill out assertive activity sheet.

SESSION 11

Set Agenda

Review Practice

A. Review and collect diaries.

B. Complete the graphs.

C. Review assertiveness skills and assignment.

Objective 1: *Begin social-skills training*

A. Learning skills for making friends.

B. Introduce idea of making a movie.

C. Develop a story with three parts.

• How to meet and begin talking to others.

• How to keep a conversation and friendship going.

• How to solve disagreements or conflicts.

Objective 2: *Establish the scenarios*
  A. Have the participants create and develop the scenarios.
  B. Offer poor examples as a means to clarify the issues.

Practice
  A. Continue to complete the diaries.
  B. Watch for a person you would like to know better.
  C. Therapists record scenarios, actors, and lines on the social-skills scenario sheet.

SESSION 12

Set Agenda

Review Practice
  A. Review diaries.
  B. Complete the graphs.
  C. Collect the diaries.
  D. Check to see what they learned about a person they want to know better.

Objective 1: *Give the participants some practice at initiating social interactions*
  A. Review progress on the movie, especially in regard to the appropriate social skills.
  B. Role-play situations from the movie (i.e., wanting to join in with a group of kids at school).

Objective 2: *Extend the participants' skills at maintaining conversations and friendships*
  A. How do you keep a conversation going?
  B. How do you end a conversation?

Practice
  A. Continue the diaries.
  B. Meet the person you want to get to know, and talk with that person.
  C. Therapists introduce and explain thought records.
  D. Therapist fills out worksheet for Session 12.

SESSION 13

Set Agenda

Review Practice
  A. Complete and discuss graphs.
  B. Discuss participants' use of assertiveness skills.
  C. Collect diaries and thought records.

Objective 1: *Practice using relaxation*

   A. Lead participants through a short relaxation exercise.

   B. Lead an imagery exercise focusing on the social situation of entering a group conversation.

Objective 2: *Resolving conflicts*

   A. Discuss conflicts, process participants' own examples.

   B. Discuss idea of "compromise."

   C. Create a list of conflicts the participants might encounter.

Objective 3: *Rehearse resolving conflicts*

   A. Pick people to role-play situations from the list of conflicts.

   B. Emphasize the following:
- Stop and relax, calm down.
- Think about what you are going to say or do before doing it.
- Think of a compromise.
- Be assertive in your suggestion.
- Negotiate.

Practice

   A. Continue making and getting to know new friends.

   B. Complete diaries.

   C. Complete thought records.

   D. Therapists fill in worksheets.

SESSION 14

Set Agenda

Review Practice

   A. Complete graphs.

   B. Discuss use of social skills.

   C. Collect thoughts record and diaries.

Objective 1: *Complete the filming*

Lead the participants through the following steps:
- Choose the situation and actors.
- Review the important points for each skill.
- Rehearse the chosen situations.
- Include planned errors with the other members offering corrective feedback.
- Choose someone to narrate and introduce the situations.
- Rehearse the narration.
- Begin filming.

Practice

   A. Complete the diaries.

   B. Complete thought records.

   C. Encourage participants to integrate the skills over the next few days.

SESSION 15

Set Agenda

Review Practice
  A. Complete graphs.
  B. Check on participants' use of social skills.
  C. Collect diaries and thought records.

Objective 1: *Extend participants' knowledge of the impact of thoughts on mood*
  A. Remind participants of the three things that affect mood.
  B. Emphasize how we have dealt with two of them:
    • Things that we do.
    • Things that happen to you.
  C. Remind participants of the example involving a noise in the house.
  D. Mistaken thoughts and emotions; tell stories involving kids and their mistaken thoughts.

Objective 2: *Introduction to a personal scientist approach*
  A. Introduce the four steps to the "personal scientist approach."
    • Catch your thoughts when you start to feel bad.
    • Write them down with a description of the situation.
    • Act like an "investigator" and test whether your thoughts were reasonable and true.
    • Come up with new thoughts that will be true and help you feel better (generation of alternatives).
  B. Summarize the four steps.

Objective 3: *Practice the personal scientist approach*
  A. Therapists role-play the examples.
  B. Role-play additional examples as needed.

Objective 4: *Apply the personal scientist approach to participants' thoughts*
  Use examples from participants' diaries.

Practice
  A. Complete thought records.
  B. Complete the diaries.
  C. Use the personal scientist approach when possible.

SESSION 16

Set Agenda

Review Practice
  Review participants' thought records and use of the personal scientist approach.

Objective 1: *Expand participants' knowledge of cognitive errors*
  Tell the group stories that illustrate the different types of processing errors.

Objective 2: *Mastery exercises*
  A. Use examples from participants' past thought records.
  B. Have participants fill out a new automatic thoughts questionnaire and discuss any improvements.
  C. Use examples from participants' automatic thoughts questionnaires to have them help each other deal with negative thoughts.
  D. Model your own thoughts when appropriate.

Objective 3: *Introduction to problem solving*
  A. Problem-solving model:
    • Identify problem.
    • Analyze the problem, "What's the problem?"
    • Generate alternative solutions and think through.
    • Choose and try an option; if it doesn't work, try another option.
  B. Present the group with examples of problem-solving.

Objective 4: *Practice problem solving*
  A. Have participants generate problem situations.
  B. Lead them through the problem-solving process.

Practice
  Continue to complete thought record, diary, and apply problem-solving.

SESSION 17

Set Agenda

Review Practice
  A. Review thought records.
  B. Have group focus on and process any problematic thoughts.
  C. Watch for dysfunctional themes or attitudes.

Objective 1: *Problem-solving mastery exercise*
  A. Review problem-solving modes.
  B. Role-play problem-solving.

Objective 2: *Introduction to attribution retraining: Consequences and causes*
  A. Explain consequences, positive and negative.
  B. Explain causes, use example about crashing noise in the night.
  C. Go over relevant cartoons.

Objective 3: *Attribution dimensions (internality–externality)*
  A. Present attribution wheel.
  B. Discuss locus of control; internal and external attributions.
  C. Use the attribution wheel to process examples provided.

Objective 4: *Review attribution concepts and describe how sad kids typically think about causes*

A. Review consequences and causes of events and their affect on feelings.
B. Discuss sad kids' tendency toward misattribution:
  • Thinks about bad or negative consequences.
  • Blames him- or herself.

Practice
A. Complete diaries.
B. Choose three events/activities from pleasant and unpleasant events schedule and write down positive causes and consequences of these.

SESSION 18

Set Agenda

Review Practice
A. Complete graphs.
B. Check to see if the parents are being helpful.

Objective 1: *Review the concept of attribution (blame) and go over homework*
A. Discuss how they monitored positive consequences.
B. Review blame and its effect on mood.

Objective 2: *Extending the concept of attributions*
A. Discuss how unhappy kids tend to think.
B. Use Nicki's depressive attributional style as an example.
C. Use "selling calendars" examples to process how what we think causes an event affects the way we feel.

Objective 3: *Attribution retraining*
A. Facilitate exercise in which participants pick situations on notecards and think of possible causes; think of at least one cause that is realistic and promotes feeling good about oneself.
B. Stress the need for causes to be viewed realistically:
  • If you fail a test it may be because of your lack of effort.
  • Use manual and Kastan items for generating more "causes."

Practice
A. Diaries.
B. Check the events in your diary and determine which are caused by you and which by other factors.

SESSION 19

Set Agenda

Review Practice
A. Complete graphs.
B. Review thought records.
C. Remind participants of the importance of continuing to work on finding negative thoughts.

Objective 1: *Establish standards in a concrete manner*
Have participants complete and score "My Standards Questionnaire—Revised" (see Appendix L).

Objective 2: *Introduction to self-evaluation*
A. Explain what the "My Standards" scores mean.
B. Process how the way you evaluate yourself affects the way you feel.

Objective 3: *Relationship of self-evaluations to ourselves*
Explain how sad kids negatively evaluate themselves.

Objective 4: *Identify an area for self improvement*
Choose, from your standards, the three most important areas for self-improvement.

Practice
A. Diaries
B. Think about your three standards and write down any more realistic standards you can think of for yourself and give your reasons for deciding to change or keep a standard.

SESSION 20

Set Agenda

Review Practice
A. Complete graphs.
B. Discuss new standards.
C. Model rational thinking and evaluate maladaptive cognitions where possible.

Objective 1: *Establish goals*
Use new standards as goals:
- Have participants designate new standards that are higher than they are presently performing.
- Get a volunteer to use his or her new standards as an example.

Objective 2: *Break the goals into subgoals*
Use the Columbus ship and karate black belt examples.

Objective 3: *Help participants to start working toward self-improvement*
Choose one goal and generate big rewards for when you accomplish it.

Practice
Diaries.
Work toward your subgoal.

SESSION 21

Review and emphasize continued use of the skills that have been learned.

APPENDIX D
Form Used for
Self-Monitoring Cognitions

THOUGHT RECORD

Remember to complete this whenever you have these feelings and to bring your booklet with you to group.

HAPPINESS

What was happening:

What I was doing:

What I was thinking:

SADNESS

What was happening:

What I was doing:

What I was thinking:

ANGRY

What was happening:

What I was doing:

What I was thinking:

APPENDIX E
Form Used for
Self-Monitoring and
Restructuring Cognitions

THOUGHT RECORD

Remember to complete this form each time that you feel sad or angry and to bring your booklet to group.

I was feeling _____

What was happening:

What I was doing:

My thoughts were:

The evidence was:

Alternative ways of thinking:
1.
2.
3.
4.
5.

What might happen:

The thought I choose to believe:

APPENDIX F
Pleasant Events Schedule for
Fourth Graders

MY DIARY

_____ 1. Someone gives me something (a gift, candy, money)

_____ 2. Someone takes me someplace special (out to eat)

_____ 3. Someone lets me know they like me or asks to be my friend

_____ 4. People tell me that they love me or kiss or hug me

_____ 5. Someone invites me to come visit them

_____ 6. Someone compliments me

_____ 7. Friends invite me to play with them

_____ 8. Not having to go to school

_____ 9. Someone invites me to a party

_____ 10. Getting a new pet

_____ 11. Friends invite me to spend the night or go to their slumber party

_____ 12. Having little or no homework to do

_____ 13. Getting to do fun things at school

_____ 14. Friends or parents help me with something

_____ 15. Getting rewarded for something I've done

_____ 16. Thinking that I am . . . (smart, pretty, strong, an American)

_____ 17. Thinking that someone loves me or cares about me

_____ 18. Thinking about doing something fun (swimming)

_____ 19. Thinking about one of my fantasies or wishes (being rich)

_____ 20. Thinking that I am good at (sports, schoolwork)

_____ 21. Thinking that my friends like me or care about me

_____ 22. Thinking about my pets, or about getting a pet

_____ 23. Thinking about nice things (rainbows, my birthday)

_____ 24. Thinking about spending time with my parents

_____ 25. Thinking about doing well in the future (getting all A's)

_____ 26. Thinking that I like or love someone (boyfriend or girlfriend)

_____ 27. Thinking about going somewhere special (Disney World)

_____ 28. Thinking that I have nice friends

_____ 29. Thinking about eating something (candy)

_____ 30. Thinking about helping people or doing something nice for them

_____ 31. Playing a team sport (football, baseball, softball, soccer)

_____ 32. Swimming

_____ 33. Spending time with, playing, or going places with my friends

_____ 34. Going to the movies or renting a movie

_____ 35. Skating

_____ 36. Watching TV

_____ 37. Eating out at a restaurant

_____ 38. Riding my bike or motorcycle or three-wheeler

_____ 39. Eating something I like (pizza, ice cream)

_____ 40. Traveling, going on vacation, going out of town

_____ 41. Doing something with parents, brother, sister, or cousin

_____ 42. Fishing

_____ 43. Going over to a friend's house, or having them come over to mine

_____ 44. Playing a video game

_____ 45. Having someone spend the night, spending the night at a friend's

_____ 46. Doing nature activities (camping, hiking in the woods)

_____ 47. Going to school

_____ 48. Visiting someone (relatives)

_____ 49. Drawing, painting, or some other form of art

_____ 50. Going to the mall

_____ 51. Boxing, wrestling, karate

_____ 52. Shopping

_____ 53. Running

_____ 54. Skateboarding

_____ 55. _____

_____ 56. _____

_____ 57. _____

_____ 58. _____

_____ 59. _____

_____ 60. _____

0	1	2	3	4	5	6	7	8	9	10
Worst mood ever					OK mood					Best mood ever

APPENDIX G
Pleasant Events Schedule for
Fifth Graders

MY DIARY

_____ 1. Someone takes me someplace special (out to eat, to Six Flags)
_____ 2. Someone compliments me
_____ 3. Someone gives me something (a gift, candy, money)
_____ 4. Friends ask me to go places with them
_____ 5. Friends invite me to play with them
_____ 6. My parents do fun things with me
_____ 7. Friends invite me to spend the night
_____ 8. Someone lets me know they like me
_____ 9. Someone comes to visit me (cousins, grandparents)
_____ 10. People call me on the phone and talk to me
_____ 11. My parents let me do fun things (go fishing, skating)
_____ 12. People come over to my house
_____ 13. Someone buys me new clothes
_____ 14. Someone lets me know that I'm special, or smiles at me
_____ 15. Someone invites me to come visit them
_____ 16. Someone asks me to "go with them"
_____ 17. Someone invites me to a party
_____ 18. Someone helps me when I'm in a "tight spot"
_____ 19. Judges place me 1st or 2nd on my project
_____ 20. My friends get along
_____ 21. Thinking that someone loves me
_____ 22. Thinking that I'm good at . . . (sports, schoolwork)
_____ 23. Thinking that I am . . . (smart, pretty, strong, an American)
_____ 24. Thinking about doing something fun (swimming)
_____ 25. Thinking that I have nice friends
_____ 26. Thinking about getting out of school for the summer
_____ 27. Thinking that my friends like me/care about me
_____ 28. Thinking that I like my teacher or that I have a nice teacher
_____ 29. Thinking about being complimented
_____ 30. Thinking how others think I am (smart, pretty)
_____ 31. Thinking about doing well in the future (getting all A's)
_____ 32. Thinking about things I've done well in the past (making home runs)
_____ 33. Thinking that I like or love someone (boyfriend, girlfriend)
_____ 34. Thinking about visiting someone or having them visit me
_____ 35. Thinking that I or my family has . . . (a new house, a puppy)
_____ 36. Thinking about doing something nice for someone else
_____ 37. Thinking about winning at . . . (a contest, a baseball game)

_____ 38. Thinking about getting a new pet
_____ 39. Thinking about nice things (flowers, rainbows)
_____ 40. Thinking about going somewhere special (Disney World)
_____ 41. Watching TV
_____ 42. Going to the movies or renting a movie
_____ 43. Eating out at a restaurant
_____ 44. Shopping or going to the mall
_____ 45. Spending time with, playing, or going places with my friends
_____ 46. Skating (roller-skating or ice-skating)
_____ 47. Eating something good like pizza or ice cream
_____ 48. Swimming
_____ 49. Playing softball or baseball
_____ 50. Going to school
_____ 51. Sleeping
_____ 52. Traveling, going on vacation, going out of town
_____ 53. Doing something with parents, brother, sister, or cousin
_____ 54. Visiting relatives
_____ 55. Going over to a friend's house, or having them come over to mine
_____ 56. Spending money
_____ 57. Riding my bike
_____ 58. Riding a horse
_____ 59. Drawing or painting
_____ 60. Playing with pets
_____ 61. Dancing
_____ 62. Playing board games
_____ 63. Talking on the phone
_____ 64. Reading a book
_____ 65. Playing an instrument
_____ 66. Going someplace special (Six Flags)
_____ 67. Fishing
_____ 68. Playing soccer
_____ 69. Playing video games
_____ 70. Partying
_____ 71. _____
_____ 72. _____
_____ 73. _____
_____ 74. _____
_____ 75. _____

0	1	2	3	4	5	6	7	8	9	10
Worst mood ever					OK mood					Best mood ever

APPENDIX H
Pleasant Events Schedule for Sixth Graders

MY DIARY

_____ 1. My parents take me someplace special (out to eat, to Six Flags)
_____ 2. Someone compliments me
_____ 3. Someone gives me something (a gift, candy, money)
_____ 4. Friends ask me to go places with them
_____ 5. Friends invite me to spend the night
_____ 6. My parents let me do fun things
_____ 7. Friends invite me to play with them
_____ 8. Someone lets me know they like me
_____ 9. Someone comes to visit me (cousins, grandparents)
_____ 10. People call me on the phone and talk to me
_____ 11. My parents do fun things with me
_____ 12. People come over to my house
_____ 13. Someone buys me new clothes
_____ 14. Someone lets me know that I'm special, or smiles at me
_____ 15. Someone invites me to come visit them
_____ 16. Someone asks me to "go with them"
_____ 17. Someone invites me to a party
_____ 18. Someone helps me when I'm in a "tight spot"
_____ 19. Judges place me 1st or 2nd on my project
_____ 20. My friends get along
_____ 21. Thinking that someone loves me
_____ 22. Thinking that I'm good at . . . (sports, schoolwork)
_____ 23. Thinking that I am . . . (smart, pretty, strong, an American)
_____ 24. Thinking about doing something fun (swimming)
_____ 25. Thinking that I have nice friends
_____ 26. Thinking about getting out of school for the summer
_____ 27. Thinking that my friends like me/care about me
_____ 28. Thinking that I like my teacher or that I have a nice teacher
_____ 29. Thinking about being complimented
_____ 30. Thinking how others think I am . . . (smart, pretty)
_____ 31. Thinking about doing well in the future (getting all A's)
_____ 32. Thinking about things I've done well in the past (making home runs)
_____ 33. Thinking that I like or love someone (boyfriend, girlfriend)
_____ 34. Thinking about visiting someone or having them visit me
_____ 35. Thinking that I or my family has . . . (a new house, a puppy)
_____ 36. Thinking about doing something nice for someone else

_____ 37. Thinking about winning at . . . (a contest, baseball game)
_____ 38. Thinking about getting a new pet
_____ 39. Thinking about nice things . . . (flowers, rainbows)
_____ 40. Thinking about going somewhere special (Disney World)
_____ 41. Watching TV
_____ 42. Going to the movies or renting a movie
_____ 43. Eating out at a restaurant
_____ 44. Shopping or going to the mall
_____ 45. Spending time with, playing, or going places with my friends
_____ 46. Skating
_____ 47. Eating something good like pizza or ice cream
_____ 48. Swimming
_____ 49. Playing softball or baseball
_____ 50. Going to school
_____ 51. Sleeping
_____ 52. Traveling, going on vacation, going out of town
_____ 53. Doing something with parents, brother, sister, or cousin
_____ 54. Visiting relatives
_____ 55. Going over to a friend's house, or having them come over to mine
_____ 56. Spending money
_____ 57. Riding my bike
_____ 58. Riding a horse
_____ 59. Drawing or painting
_____ 60. Playing with pets
_____ 61. Dancing
_____ 62. Playing board games
_____ 63. Talking on the phone
_____ 64. Reading a book
_____ 65. Playing an instrument
_____ 66. Going someplace special . . . (Six Flags)
_____ 67. Fishing
_____ 68. Playing soccer
_____ 69. Playing video games
_____ 70. Partying
_____ 71. _____
_____ 72. _____
_____ 73. _____
_____ 74. _____
_____ 75. _____

0	1	2	3	4	5	6	7	8	9	10
Worst mood ever					OK mood					Best mood ever

APPENDIX I
Assessment of
Pleasant Events

THINGS THAT ARE FUN TO DO

On this page you are to write down five things that are fun for you or that you enjoy doing. On the lines below, write down five fun things that you might do during a weekday or on a weekend. These could be things like watching TV, going out to eat, going to the movies, or playing with your friends. It can be anything that you like, even things like eating candy.

Think about the things that you do that make you happy or make you feel good when you are doing them. After you have thought a while write down five things. Don't worry about spelling—just do the best you can in writing them down. No one will grade or check your answers. Remember it is important to write down the things that are fun for you. They may be things that other kids don't like to do, but that is OK. After you write down five things, put an X over the face that tells how much fun you think each thing is.

If it's just OK put an X over the 😐 face.

If it's really fun or you like doing it a lot, put an X over the 😃 face.

If it's somewhere in between OK and a lot of fun, put an X over the 🙂 face.

Remember, think about the things that make you happy or feel good when you do them. After you have thought about it, write them down.

1. _____   😐 🙂 😃

2. _____   😐 🙂 😃

3. _____   😐 🙂 😃

4. _____   😐 🙂 😃

5. _____   😐 🙂 😃

APPENDIX J
Form for Graphing Pleasant
Events and Mood

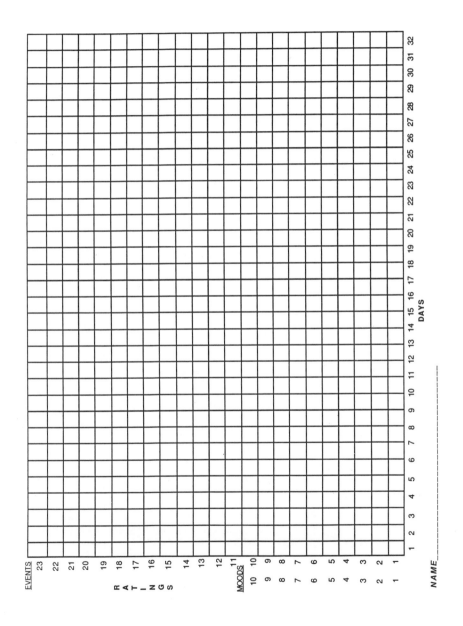

APPENDIX K
Generic
Behavioral Contract

CONTRACT

I _____ recognize that completing my
diary every day is very important and will help me learn how to enjoy myself more.
I will do the best I can to record my activities and thoughts every day and bring my
folder to our meetings.

    If you do this, I _____ agree to give you
the credit you deserve for completing your diary, and I will give you a prize at least
six of the times we meet.

_____

Group participant

_____

Group leader

APPENDIX L
My Standards
Questionnaire—Revised

MY STANDARDS QUESTIONNAIRE—R

Section 1

Please read the following 10 questions and answer them according to how you would really like to be. Tell how well you would need to do on each question to feel really good about yourself. If you could do very poorly, put an X over the 0. If you would only need to do average, put an X over the 5. And if you would have to do perfectly, put an X over the 10. If you would need to do better than average, put an X somewhere between 5 and 10. The closer to perfect you would have to be to feel really good about yourself, the closer to 10 you would place the X. If you feel satisfied with below-average performance, then you would put an X over a number between 5 and 0.

Please read each question carefully. Take your time to really think about each question, and then tell how well you need to do to be absolutely satisfied with yourself.

1. How popular do you have to be to feel really good about (absolutely satisfied with) yourself?

0	1	2	3	4	5	6	7	8	9	10
I don't					Average					The most
care if										popular
anyone										person in
likes me										school

2. How good do your grades have to be to feel really good about (absolutely satisfied with) yourself?

0	1	2	3	4	5	6	7	8	9	10
0%	30%	40%	50%	60%	70%	75%	80%	85%	90%	100%
I can fail					All C's					All A's
everything					Average					

3. How good looking do you have to be to feel really good about (absolutely satisfied with) yourself?

0	1	2	3	4	5	6	7	8	9	10
Ugly					Average					Like a model

4. How smart do you have to be to feel really good about (absolutely satisfied with) yourself?

0	1	2	3	4	5	6	7	8	9	10
Stupid					Average					Genius

5. How well behaved do you have to be to feel really good about (absolutely satisfied with) yourself?

0	1	2	3	4	5	6	7	8	9	10
I can do everything wrong					Average					Never do anything wrong

6. How athletic (good at sports) do you have to be to feel really good about (absolutely satisfied with) yourself?

0	1	2	3	4	5	6	7	8	9	10
A complete klutz										A superstar

7. How good-looking and fashionable do your clothes need to be to feel really good about (absolutely satisfied with) yourself?

0	1	2	3	4	5	6	7	8	9	10
Ragged and dirty clothes					OK					Right out of a fashion magazine

8. How funny do you have to be to feel really good about (absolutely satisfied with) yourself?

0	1	2	3	4	5	6	7	8	9	10
No sense of humor					Average					A comedian

9. How nice do you have to be to feel really good about (absolutely satisfied with) yourself?

0	1	2	3	4	5	6	7	8	9	10
Meanest person					Average					Nicest person

10. How good must your possessions (things like money, jewelry, bicycle, toys, records, stereo, etc.) be in order to feel really good about (absolutely satisfied with) yourself?

0	1	2	3	4	5	6	7	8	9	10
The worst					Average					The best

Section 2

Please read the next 10 questions and answer them according to how well your parents think you ought to do or be in each of the following areas. As you did in Section 1 with the number scale, show how well your parents think you should do or be on each question.

Read each question carefully, take your time to really think about each question, and then place an X over the number that tells how you honestly think your parents believe you ought or should be in each area.

1. How popular do your parents think you ought to be?

0	1	2	3	4	5	6	7	8	9	10

Least popular   Average   Most popular
person in school   person in school

2. What grades do your parents think you ought to make?

0	1	2	3	4	5	6	7	8	9	10

Can fail   Average,   All A's
everything   all C's

3. How good-looking do your parents think you ought to be?

0	1	2	3	4	5	6	7	8	9	10

Not at all   Average   Like a model

4. How smart do your parents think you ought to be?

0	1	2	3	4	5	6	7	8	9	10

Stupid   Average   Genius

5. How well behaved do your parents think you ought to be?

0	1	2	3	4	5	6	7	8	9	10

Can do   Average   Never do
everything   anything
wrong   wrong

6. How athletic do your parents think you ought to be?

0	1	2	3	4	5	6	7	8	9	10

Not athletic   Average   A superstar

7. How fashionable do your parents think your clothes ought to be?

0	1	2	3	4	5	6	7	8	9	10

Unfashionable   Average   Very fashionable

8. How funny do your parents think you ought to be?

0	1	2	3	4	5	6	7	8	9	10
Not funny					Average					Very funny

9. How nice do your parents think you ought to be?

0	1	2	3	4	5	6	7	8	9	10
Mean					Average					Nice always

10. How valuable do your parents think your possessions ought to be?

0	1	2	3	4	5	6	7	8	9	10
The worst					Average					The best

Section 3

Please read the next 10 questions and answer them according to how you are feeling about yourself *right now*. Remember that this set of questions refers to how you feel you are really like right now.

Again, read each question carefully, take your time to really think about each question, and then place an X over the number that tells how you honestly feel you are like *now*.

1. How popular or unpopular are you?

0	1	2	3	4	5	6	7	8	9	10
No one likes me					Average					The most popular person

2. How good are your grades?

0	1	2	3	4	5	6	7	8	9	10
I fail everything					Average grades					All A's

3. How good looking are you?

0	1	2	3	4	5	6	7	8	9	10
Ugly					Average					I look like a model

4. How smart are you?

0	1	2	3	4	5	6	7	8	9	10
Stupid					Average					Genius

5. How well behaved are you?

0	1	2	3	4	5	6	7	8	9	10
I do everything wrong					OK					I never do anything wrong

6. How athletic are you?

0	1	2	3	4	5	6	7	8	9	10
I'm a klutz					Average					I'm a superstar

7. How goodlooking are your clothes?

0	1	2	3	4	5	6	7	8	9	10
Ragged and dirty					OK					Right out of fashion magazines

8. How funny are you?

0	1	2	3	4	5	6	7	8	9	10
Not at all					Average					I'm a comedian

9. How nice are you?

0	1	2	3	4	5	6	7	8	9	10
The meanest person					Average					The nicest person

10. How good are your possessions?

0	1	2	3	4	5	6	7	8	9	10
The worst					Average					The best

Section 4

Please rank-order the following 10 things according to how important each one is to you. For example, if having good looks is most important to you, you would put a 1 in the blank next to good looks. If nice possessions are least important to you, you would put a 10 in the blank next to nice possessions.

Again, please take your time to really think about each one of the 10 things before assigning a number to each one.

____ Popularity
____ Good grades
____ Good looks
____ Intelligence
____ Good behavior
____ Athletic
____ Good-looking and fashionable clothes
____ Funny
____ Nice
____ Nice possessions (money, toys, records, etc.)

APPENDIX M
Rewards
Assessment Survey

REWARDS

PEOPLE: List two people with whom you would like to spend more time each week but don't get a chance to.

1.

2.

PLACES: List four places where you would like to spend more time but don't get a chance to.

1.   2.

3.   4.

THINGS: List four things you do not own that you would most like to have and can afford (e.g., books, records, new shoes, etc.)

1.   2.

3.   4.

List below the six foods and drinks you like best. You may also want to include items you don't get very often.

1.   2.

3.   4.

5.   6.

ACTIVITIES: List six activities you would like to do more often than you do now.

1.   2.

3.   4.

5.   6.

Now read back over your list and circle the number in front of the item in each section that you like the best.

APPENDIX N
Activity-Scheduling Form

WEEKLY ACTIVITY SCHEDULE							
date							
time	**MON**	**TUE**	**WED**	**THUR**	**FRI**	**SAT**	**SUN**
8:00							
9:00							
10:00							
11:00							
12:00							
1:00							
2:00							
3:00							
4:00							
5:00							
6:00							
7:00							
8:00							
9:00							
10:00							

APPENDIX O
Sample
Guided Imagery Exercise

We are now going to do a relaxation and imagery exercise that will start off like the other relaxation exercises we have done in previous meetings. Once you are relaxed, I will lead you through an imagery exercise that relates to what we have been talking about today—being assertive and telling someone, like a parent or close friend, that they are doing something you don't like.

Now, I want you to get comfortable in your chair and rest your hands on your legs. Close your eyes and take three deep, slow breaths. As you breathe in slowly, concentrate on the air as it fills your lungs, and as you breathe out slowly, notice the sensations of your wind rushing out through your nose and mouth. Breathe in nice and slow . . . focusing on the cool sensation of air passing in and out of your body . . . (pause about 10 seconds).

Now, I want you to clench your right fist as tight as you can, and hold it while I count down from 5 . . . focus on the tension in your fist as I begin to count . . . 5 . . . 4 . . . 3 . . . 2 . . . 1 . . . relax your fist and notice the feeling of relaxation and coolness that flows through your arm . . . focus on the feeling of relaxation that fills your arm . . . (pause about 10 seconds). Now, clench your left hand into a fist and hold it while I count down from 5 . . . focus on the tension you feel in your arm . . . 5 . . . 4 . . . 3 . . . 2 . . . 1 . . . release your fist and notice how the tension slowly leaves your arm and is replaced by a cool feeling of relaxation . . . (pause about 10 seconds). Now, hunch your shoulders so they press against your head and neck, and focus on the tension this creates as I count down from 5—5 . . . 4 . . . 3 . . . 2 . . . 1 . . . As you relax your shoulders, pay attention to the cool, soothing feelings of relaxation that run down your head, neck, and shoulders . . . (pause about 10 seconds). Hunch your shoulders again, focusing on the tension this creates as I count down from 5—5 . . . 4 . . . 3 . . . 2 . . . 1 . . . As you relax your shoulders again, focus on the feelings of relaxation that flow down your neck and through your body . . . (pause about 10 seconds).

With your eyes still closed, I now want you to imagine that you are at home, sitting in your room. You are thinking about something that one of your parents does that upsets you, something you would like to see changed. As you sit in your room, you think back to our discussion in group and how we talked about being assertive with our parents. You remember how important it is to not be nasty or disrespectful to your parents when trying to be assertive but that it is also your right to tell someone, even your parents, that they are doing something that is bothering you. You also remember the best way to tell someone they are doing something that bothers you, which is first to tell them what it is that they are doing that you don't like, how it makes you feel when they do it, and what you would like them to do instead.

As you think about these ideas and guidelines you realize how different it would be for you to be assertive with your parents, but you also realize how important it is for you to not store up your feelings. Once you have decided to approach your parents, take a minute to relax yourself and calm any anxieties you might have by taking three . . . slow . . . deep breaths . . . as you feel the relaxation from these deep breaths, I want you to think about what you are going to say to your parents when we imagine being assertive in just a minute . . . continue to take slow, deep breaths as you think about what to say when being assertive with your parents . . . (allow as much time as appears necessary for the kids to prepare themselves for the "crucial" image).

Now, as you leave your room to approach your parent, I want you to imagine that your parents will be receptive and understanding of your concerns . . . Once you are alone with your parents and as you begin the first part of your assertive statement, I want you to imagine that your parents are smiling and listening to you with an understanding look on their faces . . . as you continue to tell them about what it is that they do that bothers you, how it makes you feel, and what you would like for them to do differently, you will notice their look of concern and understanding over what you are saying . . . you are pleased to see that your parents are not getting mad as you feared they would . . . As you finish saying what you need to, you will notice a feeling of relief floating through your body . . . You may feel a sense of pride for being assertive with your parents . . . Whatever feeling you have at this moment, I want you to stay with that feeling until I finish counting down from 10—10 . . . 9 . . . 8 . . . 7 . . . 6 . . . 5 . . . 4 . . . 3 . . . 2 . . . 1 . . . OK, you can open your eyes now.

[Process how this went for the kids: Were they able to get an image? Were they able to formulate an assertive statement as we worked on in group today? How was it to be assertive with their parents in the image? Were they anxious? Did the relaxation help? Were they able to follow the instruction to image their parents as receptive? Why not? What was their feeling at the end of the imagery exercise?

Use the kids' responses to decide where they need help and provide modeling, education, and support where pertinent and necessary.]

[Be sure to use pauses throughout the relaxation and imagery exercise wherever they feel comfortable and right to do so. It is important to set a good rhythm and cadence to the exercise, not too fast and not too slow. Always try to remain aware of where the kids are at in terms of following the exercise and not getting lost and distracted. Always feel free to add to and amend this exercise to fit your particular style and the group.]

References

Achenbach, T. M., & Edelbrock, C. S. (1979). The child behavior profile: II. Boys ages 12–16 and girls aged 6–11 and 12–16. *Journal of Consulting and Clinical Psychology, 47*, 223–233.

Adam, T. A., & Stark, K. D. (1990). *Attribution style and perceived control among depressed children.* Manuscript submitted for publication.

Albert, N., & Beck, A. T. (1975). Incidence of depression in early adolescence: A prelimary study. *Journal of Youth and Adolescents, 4*, 301–307.

Amanat, E., & Butler, C. (1984). Oppressive behaviors in the families of depressed children. *Family Therapy, 11*, 65–77.

American Psychiatric Association (1987). *Diagnostic and statistical manual of mental disorders* (3rd ed., rev.). Washington, DC: Author.

Arieti, S., & Bemporad, J. R. (1980). The psychological organization of depression. *American Journal of Psychiatry, 137*, 1360–1365.

Asarnow, J. R., Carlson, G. A., & Guthrie, D. (1987). Coping strategies, self-perceptions, hopelessness, and perceived family environments in depressed and suicidal children. *Journal of Consulting and Clinical Psychology, 55*, 361–366.

Bandura, A., & Perloff, B. (1967). Relative efficacy of self-administered and externally imposed reinforcement systems. *Journal of Personality and Social Psychology, 7*, 111–116.

Bauer, A. M. (1987). A teacher's introduction to childhood depression. *The Clearing House, 61*, 81–84.

Beck, A. T., & Emery, G. (1985). *Anxiety disorders and phobias: A cognitive perspective.* New York: Basic Books.

Beck, A. T., Rush, A. J., Shaw, B. F., & Emery, G. (1979). *Cognitive therapy of depression.* New York: Guilford Press.

Beck, A. T., Ward, C. H., Mendelson, M., Mock, J., & Erbaugh, J. (1961). An inventory for measuring depression. *Archives of General Psychiatry, 4*, 561–571.

Best, L. R., & Stark, K. D. (1990). *Depressed and nondepressed children under stress: Their cognitive appraisals and coping responses.* Manuscript submitted for publication.

Bierman, K. L., Miller, C. L., & Stabb, S. D. (1987). Improving the social behavior and peer acceptance of rejected boys: Effects of social skill training with instructions and prohibitions. *Journal of Consulting and Clinical Psychology, 55,* 194–200.

Bloom, B. (1985). A factor analysis of self-report measures of family functioning. *Family Process, 24,* 225–239.

Bornstein, M. R., Bellack, A. S., & Hersen, M. (1977). Social skills training for unassertive children: A multiple baseline analysis. *Journal of Applied Behavior Analysis, 10,* 183–195.

Braswell, L., Kendall, P. C., Braith, J., Carey, M. P., & Uye, C. S. (1985). "Involvement" in cognitive–behavioral therapy with children: Process and its relationship to outcome. *Cognitive Therapy and Research, 9,* 611–630.

Brumback, R. A., Dietz-Schmidt, S. G., & Weinberg, W. A. (1977). Depression in children referred to an educational diagnostic center: Diagnosis and treatment and analysis of criteria and literature review. *Diseases of the Nervous System, 38,* 529–535.

Brumback, R. A., Jackoway, M. K., & Weinberg, W. A. (1980). Relation of intelligence to childhood depression in children referred to an educational diagnostic center. *Perceptual and Motor Skills, 50,* 11–17.

Burdock, E. L., & Hardesty, A. S. (1964). A children's behavior diagnostic inventory. *Annals of New York Academy of Science, 105,* 890–896.

Butler, L., Miezitis, S., Friedman, R., & Cole, E. (1980). The effect of two school-based intervention programs on depressive symptoms in preadolescents. *American Educational Research Journal, 17,* 111–119.

Cantwell, D. P. (1983). Depression in childhood: Clinical picture and diagnostic criteria. In D. P. Cantwell & G. A. Carlson (Eds.), *Affective disorders in childhood and adolescence: An update* (pp. 3–18). Jamaica, NY: Spectrum Publications.

Carlson, G. A., & Cantwell, D. P. (1979). A survey of depressive symptoms in a child and adolescent psychiatric population: Interview data. *Journal of the American Academy of Child Psychiatry, 18,* 587–599.

Carlson, G. A., & Cantwell, D. P. (1980). A survey of depressive symptoms, syndrome, and disorder in a child psychiatric population. *Journal of Child Psychology and Psychiatry, 21,* 19–25.

Carlson, G. A., & Cantwell, D. P. (1982). Suicidal behavior and depression in children and adolescents. *Journal of the American Academy of Child Psychiatry, 21,* 361–368.

Christ, A. E., Adler, A. G., Isacoff, M., & Gershansky, I. S. (1981). Depression: Symptoms versus diagnosis in 10,412 hospitalized children and adolescents (1957–1977). *American Journal of Psychotherapy, 35,* 400–412.

Colbert, P., Newman, B., Ney, P., & Young, J. (1982). Learning disabilities as a symptom of depression in children. *Journal of Learning Disabilities, 15,* 333–336.

Cole, D. A., & Rehm, L. P. (1986). Family interaction patterns and childhood depression. *Journal of Abnormal Child Psychology, 14*, 297–314.

Coopersmith, S. (1967). *The antecedents of self-esteem.* San Francisco: W. H. Freeman.

Drabman, R. S., Spitalnik, R. S., & O'Leary, K. D. (1973). Teaching self-control to disruptive children. *Journal of Abnormal Psychology, 82*, 10–16.

Elder, J. P., Edelstein, B. A., & Narick, M. M. (1979). Adolescent psychiatric patients: Modifying aggressive behavior with social skills training. *Behavior Modification, 3*, 161–178.

Ellis, A. (1962). *Reason and emotion in psychotherapy.* New York: Lyle Stuart.

Epstein, N., Schlesinger, S., & Dryden, W. (1988). *Cognitive–behavior therapy with families.* New York: Brunner/Mazel.

Forehand, R., Brody, G., Slotkin, J., Fauber, R., McCombs, A., & Long, N. (1988). Young adolescent and maternal depression: Assessment, interrelations, and predictors. *Journal of Consulting and Clinical Psychology, 56*, 422–426.

Frame, C., Matson, J. L., Sonis, W. A., Fialkov, M. J., & Kazdin, A. E. (1982). Behavioral treatment of depression in a prepubertal child. *Journal of Behavior Therapy and Experimental Psychiatry, 3*, 239–243.

Frommer, E., Mendelson, W. B., & Reid, M. A. (1972). Differential diagnosis of psychiatric disturbances in preschool children. *British Journal of Psychiatry, 12*, 71–74.

Fuchs, C. Z., & Rehm, L. P. (1977). A self-control behavior therapy program for depression. *Journal of Consulting and Clinical Psychology, 45*, 206–215.

Furman, E. (1974). *A child's parent dies. Studies in childhood bereavement.* New Haven: Yale University Press.

Geller, B., Chestnut, A., Miller, B., Price, C., & Yates, D. (1985). Preliminary data on DSM-III associated features of major depressive disorder in children and adolescents. *American Journal of Psychiatry, 142*, 643–644.

Goldfried, M. R., & Davison, G. C. (1976). *Clinical behavior therapy.* New York: Holt, Rinehart & Winston.

Graves, K. J., & Lahey, B. B. (1982). The effects of induced affective states on letter discrimination in disadvantaged preschool children. *Journal of Applied Developmental Psychology, 3*, 149–154.

Grossman, J. A., Poznanski, E. O., & Banegas, M. E. (1983). Lunch: Time to study family interactions. *Journal of Psychosocial Nursing and Mental Health Services, 21*, 19–22.

Haley, B. M. T., Fine, S. L., Marriage, K., Moretti, M. M., & Freeman, R. J. (1985). Cognitive bias in depression in psychiatrically disturbed children and adolescents. *Journal of Consulting and Clinical Psychology, 53*, 535–537.

Hollon, T. H. (1970). Poor school performance as a symptom of masked depression in children and adolescents. *American Journal of Psychotherapy, 24*, 258–263.

Ingram, R. E., & Kendall, P. C. (1986). Cognitive clinical psychology:

Implications of an information processing perspective. In R. E. Ingram (Ed.), *Information processing approaches to clinical psychology* (pp. 3–21). New York: Academic Press.

Kagan, J., Rosman, B. L., Day, D., Albert, J., & Phillips, W. (1964). Information processing in the child: Significance of analytic and reflective attitudes. *Psychological Monographs, 78* (Whole No. 578).

Kashani, J. H., Barbero, G. J., & Bolander, F. D. (1981). Depression in hospitalized pediatric patients. *Journal of the American Academy of Child Psychiatry, 20*, 123–134.

Kashani, J. H., Burk, J. P., & Reid, J. C. (1985). Depressed children of depressed parents. *Canadian Journal of Psychiatry, 30*, 265–269.

Kashani, J. H., & Carlson, G. A. (1987). Seriously depressed preschoolers. *American Journal of Psychiatry, 144*, 348–350.

Kashani, J., & Hakami, N. (1982). Depression in children and adolescents with malignancy. *Canadian Journal of Psychiatry, 27*, 474–477.

Kashani, J. H., Lababidi, Z., & Jones, R. S. (1982). Depression in children and adolescents with cardiovascular symptomatology: The significance of chest pain. *Journal of the American Academy of Child Psychiatry, 21*, 187–189.

Kashani, J. H., McGee, R. O., Clarkson, S. E., Andersion, J. C., Walton, L. A., Williams, A., Silva, J. C., Walton, L. A., Williams, L., & McKnew, D. H. (1983). Depression in a sample of 9-year-old children. *Archives of General Psychiatry, 40*, 1217–1227.

Kashani, J. H., & Ray, J. S. (1985). Depressive related symptoms among preschool-age children. *Child Psychiatry and Human Development, 13*, 233–238.

Kashani, J. H., Ray, J. S., & Carlson, G. A. (1984). Depression and depressive-like states in preschool-age children in a child development unit. *American Journal of Psychiatry, 141*, 1397–1402.

Kashani, J. H., & Simonds, J. F. (1979). The incidence of depression in children. *American Journal of Psychiatry, 136*, 1203–1205.

Kashani, J. H., Venzke, R., & Millar, E. A. (1981). Depression in children admitted to hospital for orthopaedic procedures. *British Journal of Psychiatry, 138*, 21–25.

Kaslow, N. J., Rehm, L. P., & Siegel, A. W. (1984). Social-cognitive and cognitive correlates of depression in children. *Journal of Abnormal Child Psychology, 12*, 605–620.

Kaslow, N. J., Stark, K. D., Printz, B., & Livingston, R. (1990). *Cognitive triad inventory for children: Development and relationship to depression and anxiety.* Manuscript submitted for publication.

Kaslow, N. J., Tanenbaum, R. L., Abramson, L. Y., Peterson, C., & Seligman, M. P. E. (1983). Problem-solving deficits and depressive symptoms among children. *Journal of Abnormal Child Psychology, 11*, 497–502.

Kaufman, K. F., & O'Leary, K. D. (1972). Reward, cost, and self-evaluation procedures for disruptive adolescents in a psychiatric hospital school. *Journal of Applied Behavior Analysis, 5*, 293–309.

Kazdin, A. E. (1981). Assessment techniques for childhood depression — A critical appraisal. *Journal of the American Academy of Child Psychiatry, 20,* 358–375.

Kazdin, A. E., Colbus, D., & Rodgers, A. (1986). Assessment of depression and diagnosis of depressive disorders among psychiatrically disturbed children. *Journal of Abnormal Child Psychology, 14,* 499–515.

Kazdin, A. E., Esveldt-Dawson, K., Sherick, R. B., & Colbus, D. (1985). Assessment of overt behavior and childhood depression among psychiatrically disturbed children. *Journal of Consulting and Clinical Psychology, 53,* 201–210.

Kazdin, A. E., French, N. H., Unis, A. S., Esveldt-Dawson, K., & Sherick, R. E. (1983). Hopelessness, depression, and suicidal intent among psychiatrically disturbed inpatient children. *Journal of Consulting and Clinical Psychology, 51,* 504–510.

Kendall, P. C. (1977). On the efficacious use of verbal self-instructional procedures with children. *Cognitive Therapy and Research, 1,* 331–341.

Kendall, P. C. (1981). Cognitive–behavioral interventions with children. In B. B. Lahey & A. E. Kazdin (Eds.), *Advances in clinical child psychology* (Vol. 4, pp. 53–90). New York: Plenum Press.

Kendall, P. C. (1985). Toward a cognitive–behavioral model of child psychopathology and a critique of related interventions. *Journal of Abnormal Child Psychology, 13,* 357–372.

Kendall, P. C., & Braswell, L. (1985). *Cognitive–behavioral therapy for impulsive children.* New York: Guilford Press.

Kendall, P. C., Cantwell, D. A., & Kazdin, A. E. (1989). Depression in children and adolescents: Assessment issues and recommendations. *Cognitive Therapy and Research, 13,* 109–146.

Kendall, P. C., Stark, K. D., & Adam, T. (1990). Cognitive deficit or cognitive distortion in childhood depression. *Journal of Abnormal Child Psychology, 18,* 255–270.

Kerr, M. M., Hoeier, T. S., & Versi, M. (1987). Methodological issues in childhood depression: A review of the literature. *American Journal of Orthopsychiatry, 57,* 193–198.

Koeppen, A. S. (1974). Relaxation training for children. *Elementary School Guidance and Counseling, 9,* 14–21.

Kovacs, M. (1981). Rating scales to assess depression in school aged children. *Acta Paedopsychiatrica, 46,* 305–315.

Kovacs, M. (1983). *The Children's Depression Inventory: A self-rated depression scale for school-aged youngsters.* Unpublished manuscript, University of Pittsburgh, Pittsburgh, PA.

Kovacs, M. (1985). The natural history and course of depressive disorders in childhood. *Psychiatric Annals, 15,* 387–389.

Kovacs, M., & Beck, A. T. (1977). An empirical–clinical approach toward a definition of childhood depression. In J. G. Schulterbrandt & A. Raskin (Eds.), *Depression in childhood: Diagnosis, treatment and conceptual models* (pp. 1–25). New York: Raven Press.

Kovacs, M., Feinberg, T. L., Crouse-Novak, M. A., Paulaskos, S. L., &

Finkelstein, R. (1984). Depressive disorders in childhood: A longitudinal prospective study of characteristics and recovery. *Archives of General Psychiatry, 41*, 229–237.

Kovacs, M., Feinberg, T. L., Crouse-Novak, M. A., Paulaskas, S. L., Pollock, M., & Finkelstein, R. (1984). Depressive disorders in childhood: II. A longitudinal study of the risk for a subsequent major depression. *Archives of General Psychiatry, 41*, 643–649.

Lang, M., & Tisher, M. (1978). *Children's Depression Scale*. Victoria, Australia: The Australian Council for Educational Research.

Laurent, J. L. (1989). *Anxiety and depression during childhood: A test of the cognitive specificity hypothesis*. Unpublished Doctoral Dissertation, University of Texas.

Lefkowitz, M. M., & Tesiny, E. P. (1985). Depression in children: Prevalence and correlates. *Journal of Consulting and Clinical Psychology, 53*, 647–656.

Leon, G. R., Kendall, P. O., & Garber, J. (1980). Depression in children: Parent, teacher and child perspectives. *Journal of Abnormal Child Psychology, 8*, 221–235.

Lewinsohn, P. M., & Graf, M. (1973). Pleasant activities and depression. *Journal of Consulting and Clinical Psychology, 41*, 261–268.

Lewinsohn, P. M., Sullivan, J. M., & Grosscup, S. J. (1980). Changing reinforcing events: An approach to the treatment of depression. *Psychotherapy: Theory, Research and Practice, 17*, 322–334.

Ling, W., Oftedal, G., & Weinberg, W. (1970). Depressive illness in childhood presenting as severe headaches. *American Journal of Diseases of Children, 120*, 122–124.

Linn, J. L., & Stark, K. D. (1990). *Childhood depression and social skills disturbances*. Manuscript submitted for publication.

Lobovits, D. A., & Handal, P. J. (1985). Childhood depression: Prevalence using DSM-III criteria and validity of parent and child depression scales. *Journal of Pediatric Psychology, 10*, 45–54.

Mahoney, M. J., & Arnkoff, D. B. (1978). Cognitive and self-control therapies. In S. L. Garfield & A. E. Bergin (Eds.), *Handbook of psychotherapy and behavior change* (2nd ed., pp. 689–722). New York: Wiley.

Masters, J. C., Barden, R. C., & Ford, M. E. (1979). Affective states, expressive behaviors, and learning in children. *Journal of Personality and Social Psychology, 37*, 380–390.

Matson, J. L., Rotatori, A. F., & Helsel, W. J. (1983). Development of a rating to measure social skills in children: The Matson Evaluation of Social Skills with Youngsters (MESSY). *Behavioral Research and Therapy, 41*, 335–340.

McGee, R., Anderson, J., Williams, S., & Silva, P. A. (1986). Cognitive correlates of depressive symptoms in 11-year-old children. *Journal of Abnormal Child Psychology, 14*, 517–524.

Meichenbaum, D. (1977). *Cognitive–behavior modification*. New York: Plenum Press.

Meichenbaum, D., & Goodman, J. (1971). Training impulsive children to talk to themselves. A means of developing self-control. *Journal of Abnormal Psychology, 77*, 115–126.

Moos, R. H., & Moos, B. S. (1981). *Family environment scale manual.* Palo Alto, CA: Consulting Psychologist Press.

Moyal, B. R. (1977). Locus of control, stimulus appraisal, and depressive symptoms in children. *Journal of Consulting and Clinical Psychology, 45*, 951–952.

Nowicki, S., Jr., & Strickland, B. R. (1973). A locus of control scale for children. *Journal of Consulting and Clinical Psychology, 40*, 148–154.

O'Leary, S. G., & Dubey, D. R. (1979). Applications of self-control procedures by children: A review. *Journal of Applied Behavior Analysis, 12*, 449–465.

Ollendick, T. H., & Cerney, J. A. (1981). *Clinical behavior therapy with children.* New York: Plenum Press.

Petti, T. A. (1978). Depression in hospitalized child psychiatry patients: Approaches to measuring depression. *Journal of the American Academy of Child Psychiatry, 17*, 49–59.

Petti, T. A., Bornstein, M., Delamater, A., & Conner, C. K. (1980). Evaluation and multimodality treatment of a depressed prepubertal girl. *Journal of the American Academy of Child Psychiatry, 19*, 690–702.

Pfeffer, C. R. (1981). The family system of suicidal children. *American Journal of Psychotherapy, 35*, 330–341.

Pfeffer, C. R., Zuckerman, S., Plutchik, R., & Mizruchi, M. S. (1984). Suicidal behavior in normal school children: A comparison with child psychiatric inpatients. *Journal of the American Academy of Child Psychiatry, 23*, 416–423.

Piers, E. V. (1969). *Manual for the Piers–Harris Children's Self-Concept Scale.* Nashville, TN: Counselor Recordings and Tests.

Poznanski, E. O., Grossman, J. A., Buchsbaum, Y., Bonegas, M., Freeman, L., & Gibbons, R. (1984). Preliminary studies of the reliability and validity of the Children's Depression Rating Scale. *Journal of the American Academy of Child Psychiatry, 23*, 191–197.

Poznanski, E. O., Krahenbuhl, V., & Zrull, J. (1976). Childhood depression. *Journal of the American Academy of Child Psychiatry, 15*, 491–501.

Poznanski, E. O., & Zrull, J. (1970). Childhood depression: Clinical characteristics of overtly depressed children. *Archives of General Psychiatry, 23*, 8–15.

Prout, H. T., & Ferber, S. M. (1988). Analogue assessment: Traditional personality assessment measures in behavioral assessment. In E. S. Shapiro & T. R. Kratochwill (Eds.), *Behavioral assessment in schools* (pp. 322–350). New York: Guilford Press.

Puig-Antich, J. (1982). The use of RDC criteria for major affective disorder in children and adolescents. *Journal of the American Academy of Child Psychiatry, 12*, 291–293.

Puig-Antich, J., Blau, S., Marx, N., Greenhill, L. L., & Chambers, W. (1978). Prepubertal major depressive disorder: A pilot study. *Journal of the American Academy of Child Psychiatry, 17*, 695–707.

Puig-Antich, J., Lukens, E., Davies, M., Goetz, D., Brennan-Quatbrock, J., & Todak, G. (1985a). Psycho-social functioning in prepubertal major depressive disorders I: Interpersonal relationships during the depressive episode. *Archives of General Psychiatry, 42*, 500–507.

Puig-Antich, J., Lukens, E., Davies, M., Goetz, D., Brennan-Quatbrock, J., & Todak, G. (1985b). Psycho-social functioning in prepubertal major depressive disorders II: Interpersonal relationships after sustained recovery from affective episode. *Archives of General Psychiatry, 42*, 511–517.

Puig-Antich, J., & Ryan, N. (1986). *Schedule for Affective Disorders and Schizophrenia for School-Age Children.* Pittsburgh, PA: Western Psychiatric Institute and Clinic.

Rehm, L. P. (1977). A self-control model of depression. *Behavior Therapy, 8*, 787–804.

Rehm, L. P., Kaslow, N. J., & Rabin, A. S. (1987). Cognitive and behavioral targets in a self-control therapy program for depression. *Journal of Consulting and Clinical Psychology, 55*, 60–67.

Reynolds, C. R., & Richmond, B. O. (1985). *Revised Children's Manifest Anxiety Scale (RCMAS) manual.* Los Angeles: Western Psychological Services.

Reynolds, W. M. (1984). Depression in children and adolescents: Phenomenology, evaluation, and treatment. *School Psychology Review, 13*, 171–182.

Reynolds, W. M. (1986). A model for the screening and identification of depressed children and adolescents in school settings. *Professional School Psychology, 1*, 117–129.

Reynolds, W. M. (1987a). *Reynolds Adolescent Depression Scale: Professional manual.* Odessa, FL: Psychological Assessment Resources.

Reynolds, W. M. (1987b). *Child Depression Scale.* Odessa, FL: Psychological Assessment Resources.

Reynolds, W. M., & Coats, K. I. (1986). A comparison of cognitive–behavioral therapy and relaxation training for the treatment of depression in adolescents. *Journal of Consulting and Clinical Psychology, 54*, 653–660.

Reynolds, W. M., Wysopal, M., & Stark, K. D. (1984). *Epidemiology of depression in children: A preliminary investigation.* Unpublished manuscript, University of Wisconsin, Madison.

Robbins, D. R., & Alessi, N. E. (1985). Depressive symptoms and suicidal behavior in adolescents. *American Journal of Psychiatry, 142*, 588–592.

Sacks, J. L. (1977). The need for subtlety. *Psychotherapy, 14*, 434–437.

Safran, J. D., Vallis, T. M., Segal, Z. V., & Shaw, B. F. (1986). Assessment of core cognitive processes in cognitive therapy. *Cognitive Therapy and Research, 10*, 509–526.

Seligman, M. E. P., Peterson, C., Kaslow, N. J., Tanenbaum, R. L., Alloy, L. B., & Abramson, L. B. (1984). Attributional style and depressive symptoms among children. *Journal of Abnormal Psychology, 93*, 235–238.

Sellstrom, E., & Stark, K. D. (1990). Schematic processing and self-reference in childhood depression. Manuscript in preparation.

Stark, K. D. (1990). *Child and Adolescent Depression Inventory: Psychometric evaluation of a measure of depression in youth.* Manuscript submitted for publication.

Stark, K. D., Adam, T., & Best, L. (1986). *My Standards Questionnaire— Revised.* Unpublished manuscript, University of Texas, Austin.

Stark, K. D., Best, L., & McCabe, N. (1990). *Development of a depressive cognitions questionnaire for children.* Manuscript submitted for publication.

Stark, K. D., & Brookman, C. (in press). Childhood depression: Theory and family-school intervention. In M. Fine & C. Carlson (Eds.), *Handbook of family-school intervention: A systems perspective.* Orlando, FL: Grune & Stratton.

Stark, K. D., Humphrey, L. L., Crook, K., & Lewis, K. (in press). Perceived family environments of depressed and anxious children: Child's and mother's perspectives. *Journal of Abnormal Child Psychology.*

Stark, K. D., Kaslow, N. J., Hill, S. J., & Lux, G. (1990). *The assessment of depression in children: Are we assessing depression or the broad-band construct of negative affectivity?* Manuscript submitted for publication.

Stark, K. D., Kaslow, N. J., Reynolds, W. M., & Kelley, A. (1990). *Cognitive–behavioral versus traditional counseling for the treatment of depressed children in the schools.* Manuscript submitted for publication.

Stark, K. D., Kendall, P. C., & Rouse, L. (1990). *Evaluation of a multiple-gate assessment procedure for identifying depressed youths.* Manuscript submitted for publication.

Stark, K. D., Laurent, J. L., Rouse, & Printz, B. (1990). *Prevalence, symptom picture, and demographic characteristics of depression during childhood.* Manuscript submitted for publication.

Stark, K. D., Livingston, R. B., Laurent, J. L., & Cardenas, B. (1990). *Childhood depression: Relationship to academic achievement and scholastic performance.* Manuscript submitted for publication.

Stark, K. D., Reynolds, W. M., & Kaslow, N. J. (1987). A comparison of the relative efficacy of self-control therapy and a behavioral problem-solving therapy for depression in children. *Journal of Abnormal Child Psychology, 15,* 91–113.

Strauss, C. C., Lahey, B. B., & Jacobsen, R. H. (1982). The relationship of three measures of childhood depression to academic underachievement. *Journal of Applied Developmental Psychology, 3,* 375–380.

Strober, M., & Carlson, G. (1982). Bipolar illness in adolescents with major depression: Clinical, genetic, and psychopharmacologic predictors in a three-to-four year prospective follow-up investigation. *Archives of General Psychiatry, 39,* 549–555.

Tesiny, E. P., Lefkowitz, M. M., & Gordon, N. H. (1980). Childhood depression, locus of control, and school achievement. *Journal of Educational Psychology, 72,* 506–510.

Turk, D. C., & Salovey, P. (1985). Cognitive structures, cognitive processes, and cognitive–behavior modification: 1. Client Issues. *Cognitive Therapy and Research, 9,* 1–18.

Turkewitz, H., O'Leary, K. D., & Ironsmith, M. (1975). Generalization and maintenance of appropriate behavior through self-control. *Journal of Consulting and Clinical Psychology, 43*, 577–583.

Vincenzi, H. (1987). Depression and reading ability in sixth-grade children. *Journal of School Psychology, 25*, 155–160.

Vosk, B., Forehand, R., Parker, J. B., & Rickard, K. (1982). A multimethod comparison of popular and unpopular children. *Developmental Psychology, 18*, 571–575.

Weinberg, W. A., Rutman, J., Sullivan, L., Penich, E. C., & Dietz, S. G. (1973). Depression in children refered to an educational diagnostic center: Diagnosis and treatment. *Journal of Pediatrics, 83*, 1065–1072.

Weller, E. B., & Weller, R. A. (1985). Clinical aspects of childhood depression. *Psychiatric Annals, 15*, 368–374.

Wirt, R. D., Lachar, D., Klinedienst, J., & Seat, P. D. (1977). *Multidimensional description of child personality: A manual for the Personality Inventory for Children.* Los Angeles: Western Psychological Services.

Wolfe, V. V., Finch, A. J., Saylor, C. F., Blount, R. L., Pallmeyer, T. P., & Carek, D. J. (1987). Negative affectivity in children: A multitrait/multimethod investigation. *Journal of Consulting and Clinical Psychology, 55*, 245–250.

Zeiss, A. M., Lewinsohn, P. M., & Munoz, R. F. (1979). Nonspecific improvment effects in depression using interpersonal skills training, pleasant activity schedules, or cognitive training. *Journal of Consulting and Clinical Psychology, 47*, 427–439.

Index